Diabetes/Kidney/Heart Disease

Editors

SILVI SHAH
CHARUHAS V. THAKAR

CARDIOLOGY CLINICS

www.cardiology.theclinics.com

August 2019 • Volume 37 • Number 3

ELSEVIER

1600 John F. Kennedy Boulevard • Suite 1800 • Philadelphia, Pennsylvania, 19103-2899

http://www.theclinics.com

CARDIOLOGY CLINICS Volume 37, Number 3
August 2019 ISSN 0733-8651, ISBN-13: 978-0-323-68121-6

Editor: Stacy Eastman
Developmental Editor: Laura Kavanaugh

Cardiology Clinics (ISSN 0733-8651) is published quarterly by Elsevier Inc., 360 Park Avenue South, New York, NY 10010-1710. Months of issue are February, May, August, and November. Business and Editorial Offices: 1600 John F. Kennedy Blvd., Ste. 1800, Philadelphia, PA 19103-2899. Customer Service Office: 3251 Riverport Lane, Maryland Heights, MO 63043. Periodicals postage paid at New York, NY and additional mailing offices. Subscription prices are $349.00 per year for US individuals, $672.00 per year for US institutions, $100.00 per year for US students and residents, $432.00 per year for Canadian individuals, $843.00 per year for Canadian institutions, $466.00 per year for international individuals, $843.00 per year for international institutions and $220.00 per year for Canadian and international students/residents. To receive student/resident rate, orders must be accompanied by name of affiliated institution, data of term, and the *signature* of program/residency coordinator on institution letterhead. Orders will be billed at individual rate until proof of status is received. Foreign air speed delivery is included in all *Clinics* subscription prices. All prices are subject to change without notice. **POSTMASTER:** Send address changes to *Cardiology Clinics*, Elsevier Health Sciences Division, Subscription Customer Service, 3251 Riverport Lane, Maryland Heights, MO 63043. **Customer Service: 1-800-654-2452 (U.S. and Canada); 314-447-8871 (outside U.S. and Canada). Fax: 314-447-8029. E-mail: journalscustomerservice-usa@ elsevier.com (for print support); journalsonlinesupport-usa@elsevier.com (for online support).**

Reprints. For copies of 100 or more, of articles in this publication, please contact the Commercial Reprints Department, Elsevier Inc., 360 Park Avenue South, New York, NY 10010-1710. Tel.: 212-633-3874; Fax: 212-633-3820; E-mail: reprints@elsevier.com.

Cardiology Clinics is also published in Spanish by McGraw-Hill Interamericana Editores S. A., P.O. Box 5-237, 06500, Mexico D. F., Mexico; in Portuguese by Reichmann and Alfonso Editores Rio de Janeiro, Brazil; and in Greek by Dimitrios P. Lagos, 8 Pondon Street, GR115-28 Ilissia, Greece.

Cardiology Clinics is covered in *MEDLINE/PubMed (Index Medicus), Excerpta Medica, The Cumulative Index to Nursing and Allied Health Literature* (CINAHL).

Contributors

JAMES E. NOVAK, MD, PhD, FACP, FASN, FNKF
Program Director, Nephrology Fellowship, Division of Nephrology, Henry Ford Hospital, Professor, Wayne State University, Detroit, Michigan

NIRALEE PATEL, MD
Division of Nephrology, Icahn School of Medicine at Mount Sinai, New York, New York

MAX REIF, MD
Professor of Medicine, University of Cincinnati Medical Center, Cincinnati, Ohio

FLORENCE ROTHENBERG, MS, MD, FACC
Associate Professor of Internal Medicine and Cardiovascular Diseases, University of Cincinnati, Cincinnati VA Medical Center, Cincinnati, Ohio

JACK RUBINSTEIN, MD
University of Cincinnati, Cincinnati, Ohio

PAGE V. SALENGER, MD
Medical Director, Home Therapies, DCI, Nashville, Tennessee

DAREK SANFORD, MD
University of Cincinnati, Cincinnati, Ohio

SYDNEY SCHACHT, DO
Department of Internal Medicine, University of Cincinnati Medical Center, University of Cincinnati, Cincinnati, Ohio

SILVI SHAH, MD, MS, FASN, FACP
Assistant Professor of Medicine, Division of Nephrology, Kidney CARE Program, University of Cincinnati, Cincinnati, Ohio

CHARUHAS V. THAKAR, MD, FASN
Division of Nephrology, Kidney CARE Program, University of Cincinnati, Renal Section, Cincinnati VA Medical Center, Cincinnati, Ohio

GEORGE THOMAS, MD, MPH, FACP, FASN
Director, Center for Blood Pressure Disorders, Department of Nephrology and Hypertension, Cleveland Clinic, Assistant Professor, Cleveland Clinic Lerner College of Medicine, Cleveland, Ohio

JILLIAN THOMPSON, DO
Department of Internal Medicine, University of Cincinnati Medical Center, University of Cincinnati, Cincinnati, Ohio

NICHOLAS WETTERSTEN, MD
Division of Cardiology, University of California, San Diego, La Jolla, California

Contents

Preface: Diabetes/Kidney/Heart Disease   ix

Silvi Shah and Charuhas V. Thakar

Cardiorenal Syndrome: Pathophysiology   251

Ujjala Kumar, Nicholas Wettersten, and Pranav S. Garimella

Cardiorenal syndrome commonly refers to the collective dysfunction of heart and kidney resulting in a cascade of feedback mechanism causing damage to both the organs and is associated with adverse clinical outcomes. The pathophysiology of cardiorenal syndrome is complex, multifactorial, and dynamic. Improving the understanding of disease mechanisms will aid in developing targeted pharmacologic and nonpharmacologic therapies for the management of this syndrome. This article discusses the various mechanisms involved in the pathophysiology of the cardiorenal syndrome.

Treatment of Cardiorenal Syndrome   267

Jack Rubinstein and Darek Sanford

The treatment of cardiorenal syndrome is as complex as the various mechanisms underlying its pathophysiology. Randomized controlled data typically focus on the treatment of heart failure with cardiac specific endpoints and a lack of worsening renal function used as a surrogate for efficacy. When heart failure is considered the inciting event, the acute state is managed with vasodilators, inotropic support, and decongestion; whereas neurohormonal axis inhibition is more commonly applied to chronic state. A recent shift in thought process regarding the interplay of cardiac and renal dysfunction suggests that renal congestion may be the primary driver of worsening renal function.

Hypertensive Emergencies: A Review of Common Presentations and Treatment Options   275

Latoya Brathwaite and Max Reif

Approximately 33% of adults in the United States have high blood pressure; approximately 1% will present with a hypertensive emergency. Hypertension emergency is typically defined as a blood pressure great than 180/120 mm Hg leading to end organ damage. However, it is important to note that an acute rise in blood pressure may also lead to end organ damage before achieving the blood pressure threshold. Therapeutic intervention should be a short-acting, easily titratable, intravenous antihypertensive medication based on the type of end-organ damage, pharmacokinetics, and comorbidities. This review focuses on presentations and treatment of hypertensive emergency.

Contrast Nephropathy Associated with Percutaneous Coronary Angiography and Intervention   287

James E. Novak and Richa Handa

Contrast nephropathy (CN) is acute kidney injury (AKI) that occurs within 24 to 72 hours of iodinated contrast medium (ICM) administration. Mechanisms of CN include hyperviscosity, free radical formation, and renal medullary oxygen supply/demand mismatch. Although risk factors for CN have been identified, it remains uncertain whether ICM causes or is simply associated with AKI. The cornerstones of CN prevention are using low-osmolal ICM, intravenous hydration, and statins, especially in patients with chronic kidney disease. With appropriate CN risk mitigation, coronary angiography and intervention should not be routinely withheld from patients with acute coronary syndromes.

Acute Kidney Injury, Heart Failure, and Health Outcomes   **297**

Prakash S. Gudsoorkar and Charuhas V. Thakar

Acute kidney injury in acute decompensated heart failure leads to increased readmissions regardless of being transient or sustained at the time of discharge. Timely identification of acute kidney injury and worsening heart failure in patients with acute decompensated heart failure is of utmost importance to optimize different components of heart failure treatment. Acute kidney injury is a strong predictor of poor outcomes and early death in patients with pulmonary artery hypertension and acute right-sided heart failure. Extracorporeal ultrafiltration should not be used as an initial or alternative to diuretic therapy. It should be reserved for diuretic-resistant individuals.

Hypertension Management in Chronic Kidney Disease and Diabetes: Lessons from the Systolic Blood Pressure Intervention Trial   **307**

George Thomas

Based on observational and clinical trials, formulation of hypertension guidelines began in 1977. Successive guideline reports recommended lower blood pressure goals, with emphasis shifting to treatment of systolic hypertension. In 2013, responsibility for hypertension guidelines was assigned to the American College of Cardiology and the American Heart Association. The new hypertension guideline was published in 2017, and the Systolic Blood Pressure Intervention Trial (SPRINT) informed many of the recommendations in the new guidelines. This article describes the SPRINT study results and the new guideline recommendations regarding hypertension management and blood pressure goals, with emphasis on chronic kidney disease and diabetes.

Sudden Cardiac Death in End-Stage Renal Disease   **319**

Page V. Salenger

The challenge presented by sudden cardiac death in dialysis patients is to better define risk factors and delineate multiple etiologies. Only then can therapy be tailored to the highest risk patients and the incidence of sudden cardiac death be reduced. This article details the many possible etiologies and presents a brief overview of more recent research that may in the future prove of great benefit in improving the mortality of our patients with end-stage renal disease.

Apolipoprotein L1, Cardiovascular Disease and Hypertension: More Questions than Answers   **327**

Niralee Patel and Girish N. Nadkarni

Ethnic disparities in health outcomes exist among multiple complex diseases especially cardiovascular disease, hypertension, and kidney disease. Recent discoveries in genetics have taught us that these disparities go beyond environmental and socioeconomic factors. The discovery of ethnic-specific risk variants in the Apolipoprotein L1 (*APOL1*) gene on chromosome 22 seen only in individuals of recent

African ancestry explains a large proportion of kidney disease disparities. In addition, recent large-scale genotype-phenotype association studies have identified associations with cardiovascular disease and hypertension. This review aims to review the recent literature in this field and point toward future directions for research.

Novel Antidiabetic Therapies and Cardiovascular Risk Reduction: The Role of the Noninferiority Trial   335

Jillian Thompson, Sydney Schacht, and Florence Rothenberg

Diabetes is a major risk factor for cardiovascular disease, yet until now treatments for diabetes had only a modest impact on cardiovascular events. New interventions for patients with type 2 diabetes mellitus (oral empagliflozin and injectable liraglutide) are associated with unprecedented reductions in composite cardiovascular outcomes that seem disproportionate to the impact on glycated hemoglobin. This review examines in detail the recent trials that arrived at these conclusions, limitations of these studies, and how these outcomes may influence patient management in the future.

Hypertensive Disorders of Pregnancy   345

Silvi Shah and Anu Gupta

Hypertensive disorders of pregnancy are common and contribute inordinately to maternal and fetal morbidity and mortality. Although not completely understood, recent clinical trials have provided important insights into pathogenesis of preeclampsia. Preeclampsia is considered a systemic disease with generalized endothelial dysfunction and risk of future cardiovascular disease. This review revisits the definitions and classifications of hypertensive disorders of pregnancy; discusses updates on pathophysiology, prevention, and early prediction of preeclampsia; reviews current management guidelines; and discusses potential risks and benefits associated with treatment. Improvement in management and outcomes of women with hypertensive disorders of pregnancy seems in sight in the near future.

CARDIOLOGY CLINICS

FORTHCOMING ISSUES

November 2019
Cardio-Oncology
Monika Jacquelina Leja, *Editor*

February 2020
Aortic Valve Disease
Marie-Annick Clavel and Philippe Pibarot,
Editors

RECENT ISSUES

May 2019
Atrial Fibrillation in Heart Failure
Benjamin Steinberg and Jonathan Piccini,
Editors

February 2019
Hypertrophic Cardiomyopathy
Julio A. Panza and Srihari S. Naidu, *Editors*

SERIES OF RELATED INTEREST

Cardiac Electrophysiology Clinics
Heart Failure Clinics
Interventional Cardiology Clinics

THE CLINICS ARE AVAILABLE ONLINE!
Access your subscription at:
www.theclinics.com

Preface
Diabetes/Kidney/Heart Disease

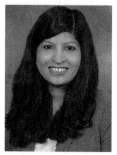 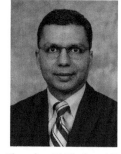

Silvi Shah, MD, MS   Charuhas V. Thakar, MD
Editors

Cardiovascular disease is the leading cause of morbidity and mortality in patients with kidney disease in the United States. The risk of cardiovascular events increases with progression of kidney disease, and significant resources are spent in health care in treating kidney and cardiovascular disease disorders. The current issue of *Cardiology Clinics* aims to bridge the gap between the 2 specialties of nephrology and cardiology. Each article comprehensively summarizes various important concepts of heart and kidney connection, including pathophysiology and management of cardiorenal syndrome, contrast-induced nephropathy, the role of novel antidiabetic therapies in cardiovascular risk reduction, apolipoprotein L1 (APOL1) in cardiovascular disease, hypertensive emergencies, and management of hypertension, with an emphasis on chronic kidney disease, diabetes, and pregnancy. We believe that the current issue of *Cardiology Clinics* will benefit the health care community in optimizing patient care and determining best practices in managing kidney in cardiovascular disease disorders.

Undoubtedly, the efforts of various clinical investigators and scientists have resulted in significant advancement in our understanding of cardiorenal syndrome. Nearly 2 decades earlier, Claudio Ronco and colleagues described 5 types of cardiorenal syndrome defined by a complex pathophysiologic disorder of the heart

and kidneys, whereby acute or chronic dysfunction in 1 organ perpetuates acute or chronic dysfunction in the other organ. Acute kidney injury is common in patients with acute and chronic heart failure and is associated not only with adverse outcomes of higher hospitals readmissions and mortality but also with higher resource utilization. Even though diuretics and extracorporeal ultrafiltration remain the cornerstone of therapy for management of volume overload in patients with heart failure, therapies at improving outcomes in this population have met with minimal success. The role of nonconventional biomarkers in diagnosing kidney disease in heart failure is still being evaluated, and hence, a gap of knowledge still remains, surely to be filled by the unrelenting progress of translational research.

This issue attempts to address several diverse yet clinically relevant areas and sheds light on directions of future investigations. For instance, (i) risk stratification for contrast-induced nephropathy is an area of special focus, since cardiac catheterization in certain patients with acute coronary syndrome is considered to save heart at the expense of kidneys; (ii) although, in recent years, health care providers have improved their understanding of hypertensive emergencies, the association of APOL1 with cardiovascular disease and hypertension still remains an open

Cardiol Clin 37 (2019) ix–x
https://doi.org/10.1016/j.ccl.2019.04.011
0733-8651/19/© 2019 Published by Elsevier Inc.

question; (iii) what are the new guideline recommendations regarding hypertension management and blood pressure goal in patients with chronic kidney disease and diabetes with recent clinical evidence?; (iv) what is the appropriate blood pressure goal in pregnant women?; and (v) what is the role of sodium-glucose cotransporter-2 inhibitors in reducing cardiovascular risk in patients with diabetes? Many of these questions have been answered, and a few still remain due to ongoing disagreements or uncertainties.

In overseeing the development of the "Diabetes/Kidney/Heart Disease" issue of *Cardiology Clinics*, we have tried to give a comprehensive perspective on the content of the articles, which includes perspective from a cardiologist and a nephrologist. The reader, therefore, should find a coordinated approach to the evaluation and initial management of patients presenting with disorders of heart and kidney. We believe that all health care providers will benefit from the content and will gain additional perspective from the nephrology specialty. We thank the authors of this "Diabetes/Kidney/Heart Disease" issue of *Cardiology Clinics* for their invaluable contribution to the existing literature of the kidney and heart connection.

Silvi Shah, MD, MS
Division of Nephrology
Kidney C.A.R.E Program
University of Cincinnati
231 Albert Sabin Way
Cincinnati, OH 45267, USA

Charuhas V. Thakar, MD
Division of Nephrology
Kidney C.A.R.E Program
University of Cincinnati
231 Albert Sabin Way
Cincinnati, OH 45267, USA

Renal Section
Cincinnati VA Medical Center
Cincinnati, OH 45220, USA

E-mail addresses:
shah2sv@ucmail.uc.edu (S. Shah)
thakarcv@ucmail.uc.edu (C.V. Thakar)

Cardiorenal Syndrome
Pathophysiology

Ujjala Kumar, MD, MPH[a], Nicholas Wettersten, MD[b], Pranav S. Garimella, MD, MPH[a],*

KEYWORDS

- Cardiorenal • Venous congestion • Intra-abdominal pressure • RAAS • Oxidative stress
- Inflammatory mediators • Uremic toxins

KEY POINTS

- Cardiorenal syndrome (CRS) is a term that commonly refers to the collective dysfunction of heart and kidneys causing a cascade of feedback mechanisms and resulting in damage to both the organs.
- Multiple mechanisms (hemodynamic, neurohormonal, inflammatory, and oxidative stress) are involved in the pathophysiology of CRS.
- In CRS, the renin-angiotensin-aldosterone system and sympathetic nervous system activation leads to salt avidity and volume overload.
- Venous congestion and increased intra-abdominal pressure play an important role in the pathophysiology of CRS.
- The role of creatinine and novel biomarkers for diagnosing kidney disease in the setting of heart failure needs to be further evaluated.

INTRODUCTION

The earliest mention of the term cardiorenal syndrome (CRS) came about from a 2004 National Heart, Lung, and Blood Institute Working Group conference evaluating the interaction between the heart and kidney.[1] The term is commonly used to refer to the collective dysfunction of the heart and kidneys resulting in a cascade of feedback mechanisms causing damage to both organs. Previously proposed definitions of CRS stressed the effects of a diseased heart on causing dysfunction of the kidney, with heart failure (HF) being the prototypical cardiovascular disease leading to kidney dysfunction from CRS. However, it is now recognized that either the heart or the kidney can be the primary source of insult. Although the term CRS is often used globally to address the pathophysiologic interaction between the two organs, a recent classification of CRS proposed by the seventh Acute Dialysis Quality Initiate consensus conference has divided the syndromes into those that are cardiorenal (**Fig. 1**), referring to when cardiac dysfunction leads to kidney dysfunction, and those that are renocardiac (**Fig. 2**), referring to when primary kidney dysfunction leads to cardiac dysfunction.[2,3] These syndromes are further classified based on their acuity and the presence of a systemic (noncardiac, nonrenal) illness that may play a role in the pathophysiology (**Fig. 3**). However, often the causal relationship (cardiorenal vs renocardiac) may not be ascertainable when risk factors like diabetes, hypertension, and atherosclerosis affect the function of both organs in parallel, leading to a common clinical picture.[4,5]

Disclosure: There are no financial conflicts of interest to disclose. However, this work was supported by NIDDK grant K23 DK114556 to P.S. Garimella and T32DK104717 to U. Kumar.

[a] Division of Nephrology-Hypertension, University of California San Diego, 9500 Gilman Drive# 9111H, La Jolla, CA 92093-9111, USA; [b] Division of Cardiology, University of California San Diego, 9434 Medical Center Drive, La Jolla, CA 92037, USA
* Corresponding author.
E-mail address: pgarimella@ucsd.edu

Cardiol Clin 37 (2019) 251–265
https://doi.org/10.1016/j.ccl.2019.04.001

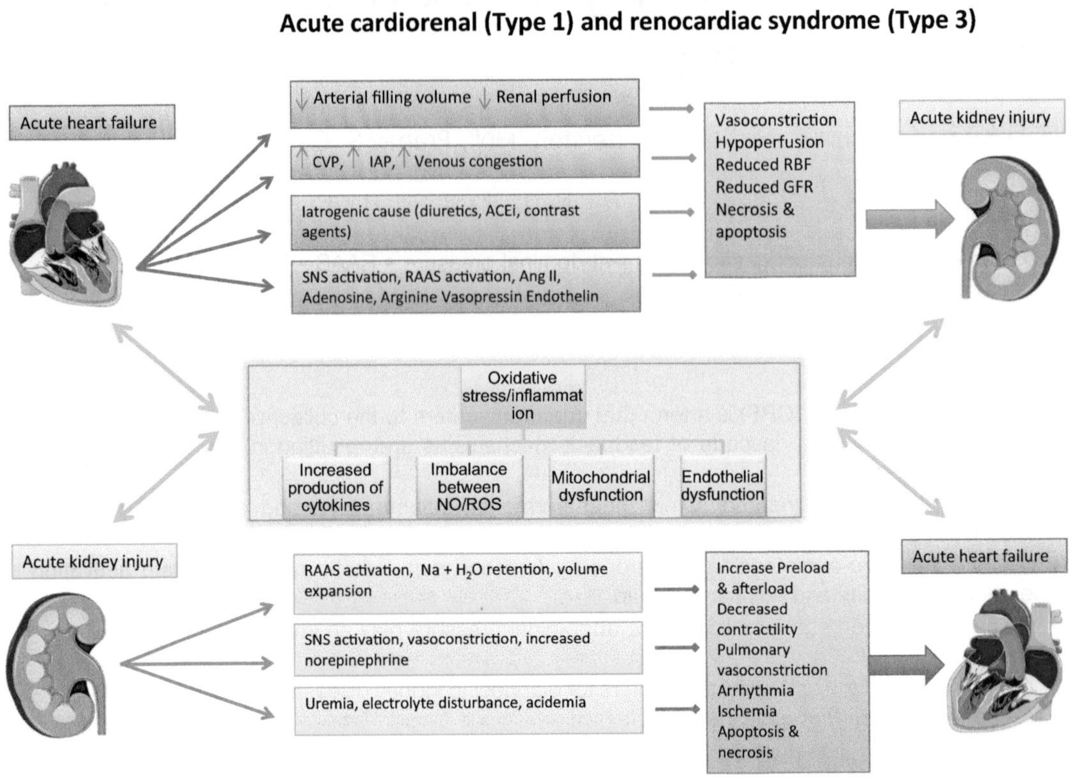

Acute cardiorenal (Type 1) and renocardiac syndrome (Type 3)

Fig. 1. Pathophysiologic interaction in acute cardiorenal syndrome (type 1) and acute renocardiac syndrome (type 3). ACEi, angiotensin-converting enzyme inhibitor; CVP, central venous pressure; GFR, glomerular filtration rate; IAP, intra-abdominal pressure; RAAS, renin-angiotensin-aldosterone system; RBF, renal blood flow; ROS, reactive oxygen species; SNS, sympathetic nervous system.

Given the aging population, longer cumulative exposure to common risk factors, including hypertension, obesity, diabetes, and vascular disorders, and advances in medical therapy, procedures, and devices to assist patients with HF live longer, the prevalences of chronic kidney disease (CKD) and HF are likely to continue to increase.[6,7] It is hence important to understand the various mechanisms involved in the propagation of this syndrome. This article reviews the role of the heart and kidney in the development of different CRSs, and the interplay between the complex pathophysiologic pathways resulting in vicious cycle and end-organ damage.

EVALUATING CHANGE IN KIDNEY FUNCTION

Acute kidney injury (AKI) refers to an abrupt reduction of kidney function, resulting in the retention of the urea and other nitrogenous toxins, dysregulation of the electrolytes, and retention of extracellular volume. Several consensus definitions of AKI have been established using serum creatinine level and urine output to accurately identify the

patients with AKI in clinical settings as well as in epidemiologic and outcomes studies. The Kidney Disease: Improving Global Outcomes (KDIGO)[8] definition is currently the most commonly used and is defined as follows:

- Increase in serum creatinine level by greater than or equal to 0.3 mg/dL ($\geq$26.5 μmol/L) in a 48-hour period
- Increase in serum creatinine level to greater than or equal to 1.5 times baseline, which is known or presumed to have occurred within the prior 7 days
- Urine volume less than 0.5 mL/kg/h for 6 hours

The KDIGO criteria further stage AKI into 3 categories, as shown in **Table 1**.[8]

However, there are concerns about the utility of serum creatinine as a biomarker to diagnose AKI in persons with HF. Volume overload in the setting of HF may lead to seemingly normal or even low creatinine value. Unmasking the effect of dilution is often mistaken for AKI, leading to a decrease in dose or cessation of diuretics, which may be

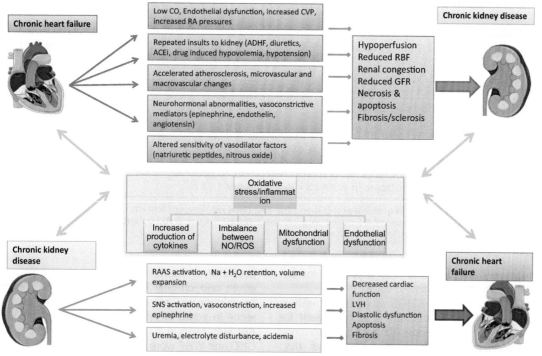

Chronic cardiorenal (Type 2) and renocardiac syndrome (type 4)

Fig. 2. Pathophysiology of chronic cardiorenal syndrome (type 2) and chronic renocardiac syndrome (type 4).

inappropriate.[9] Patients with acute decompensated HF (ADHF) who are left with residual congestion have increased mortality and risk of readmission.[10,11]

Most patients with ADHF present with signs and symptoms of fluid overload and are treated with diuretic therapy.[12] Up to 33% of patients may have an increase in creatinine level during treatment.[5] Although this increase can meet KDIGO criteria for AKI, the cardiology literature often refers to this as worsening renal function (WRF) because it is not clear that there is evidence of kidney injury and often the increase is thought to be a hemodynamic effect.[7] Further confounding the issue are a decreased muscle mass and protein intake and increased levels of inflammation, which are common in advanced HF and may be exacerbated by acute deteriorations in heart and kidney function and frequent hospitalizations. Alterations in these parameters may result in changes in serum creatinine level, leading to errors in estimated glomerular filtration rate (eGFR) and thus

Fig. 3. Types of cardiorenal syndrome.

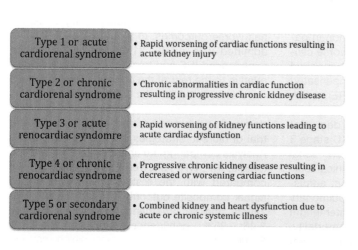

Type 1 or acute cardiorenal syndrome	• Rapid worsening of cardiac functions resulting in acute kidney injury
Type 2 or chronic cardiorenal syndrome	• Chronic abnormalities in cardiac function resulting in progressive chronic kidney disease
Type 3 or acute renocardiac syndomre	• Rapid worsening of kidney functions leading to acute cardiac dysfunction
Type 4 or chronic renocardiac syndrome	• Progressive chronic kidney disease resulting in decreased or worsening cardiac functions
Type 5 or secondary cardiorenal syndrome	• Combined kidney and heart dysfunction due to acute or chronic systemic illness

Table 1
KDIGO staging of acute kidney injury

Stage	Serum Creatinine	Urine Output
1	1.5–1.9 times baseline OR ≥0.3 mg/dl (≥26.5 μmol/1) increase	<0.5 ml/kg/h for 6–12 h
2	2.0–2.9 times baseline	<0.5 ml/kg/h for ≥12 h
3	3.0 times baseline OR Increase in serum creatinine to ≥4.0 mg/dl (≥353.6 μmol/l) OR Initiation of renal replacement therapy OR, In patients <18 y, decrease in eGFR to <35 ml/min per 1.73 m²	<0.3 ml/kg/h for ≥24 h OR Anuria for ≥12 h

Abbreviations: eGFR, estimated glomerular filtration rate; RRT, renal replacement therapy.

Reprinted from Kidney International Supplements, Volume 2, Issue 2, Section 2: AKI Definition, Page 8. Copyright 2012. With permission from Elsevier.

negatively affecting care and outcomes for patients with HF and kidney disease.

CKD is defined by KDIGO as an abnormality in kidney function or structure that is present for greater than 3 months. The most common functional abnormality is an eGFR less than 60 mL/min/1.73 m² with or without the presence of persistent kidney damage (albumin to creatinine ratio of greater than 30 mg/g, urine sediment abnormalities, tubular dysfunction, history of kidney transplant).[13] Recent KDIGO guidelines have classified CKD based on glomerular filtration rate (GFR), and degree of albuminuria (A1<30 mg/g; A2 30–300 mg/g; A3>300 mg/g).

Although albuminuria is often thought of in the context of CKD, this is not always the case in patients with CRS. In the setting of HF and CRS, albuminuria may not be a product of CKD but an effect of cardiac dysfunction.[14–16]

EPIDEMIOLOGY

Impairment in kidney function is common in patients with HF and is associated with worse clinical outcomes than in persons without impaired kidney function. In the Acute Decompensated Heart Failure National Registry (ADHERE), which included more than 105,000 patients admitted with ADHF, 91% of patients had some degree of renal dysfunction, with 64% having CKD stage 3 or higher. Patients with more severe renal dysfunction had worse in-hospital clinical outcomes (need for mechanical ventilation, admission to an intensive care unit, cardiopulmonary resuscitation, new-onset dialysis), greater length of hospital stay, and greater in-hospital mortality. Overall, eGFR was found to be an independent

predictor of mortality.[17] In a meta-analysis of acute and chronic HF populations, the overall prevalence of CKD was 49% (with higher prevalence in acute HF [53%] vs chronic HF [42%]). AKI was seen in 23% to 35% of patients. Both CKD and WRF were associated with significantly increased mortality risk.[18]

In addition to the lack of a consensus definition of AKI in the setting of HF, the clinical significance of these changes has recently been brought into question. Specifically, the context in which renal function changes needs to be considered when deciding on whether it is truly a deleterious state. Recent studies have shown that AKI occurring in response to diuretic treatment is associated with symptomatic improvement and signs of decongestion seems to be associated with improved outcomes, whereas AKI without appropriate response to therapy is associated with worse outcomes.[19–21]

In addition, other studies have shown that improvement in renal function (IRF) in ADHF has worse outcomes. In a study of 900 patients admitted with ADHF, 31.4% of the population experienced IRF and had an increased mortality relative to the rest of the cohort.[22] Similar results were seen in the Diuretic Optimization Strategies Evaluation (DOSE), which was a multicenter, randomized, double-blind, and placebo-controlled trial of diuretic strategies in patients with ADHF. Analysis comparing the changes in renal function (stable, IRF, WRF) showed that patients with IRF compared with the rest of the cohort had a higher composite outcome of death, rehospitalization, and an emergency visits (hazard ratio, 2.46; 95% confidence interval, 1.54–3.93; P<.001).[23]

Serum creatinine has remained the most widely measured marker of kidney function, but it evaluates the function of the glomerulus and does not necessarily reflect tubular function or injury. This limitation has led to several novel biomarkers being evaluated in the diagnosis of AKI, specifically from tubular damage.[24,25] A recent study investigated a panel of kidney tubular injury biomarkers, including neutrophil gelatinase-associated lipocalin (NGAL), N-acetyl-β-D-glucosaminidase (NAG), and kidney injury molecule 1 (KIM-1) in patients with ADHF with and without WRF.[26] Kidney tubular injury biomarkers did not seem to have an association with WRF in the context of aggressive diuresis of patients with ADHF. These data suggest that the increases in creatinine levels seen in the course of diuresis during ADHF may not be AKI, thus bringing into the question the sensitivity of serum creatinine to diagnose true kidney injury. Therapies such as ultrafiltration for HF have fallen out of favor, given the seeming lack of benefit and increased risk of AKI (using serum creatinine),[27] but whether this reflects true tubular damage needs to be confirmed using these novel biomarkers.

MECHANISM OF DISEASE PROCESS

Some of the difficulties in defining, researching, and treating CRS stem from the fact that multiple different pathophysiologic processes are involved (hemodynamic, hormonal, inflammatory). Thus, although it is more simplistic to consider individual pathophysiologic processes, these individual processes must be recognized as one portion of a larger multifaceted and complex pathophysiology (**Table 2**). In addition, the significance and impact of each process varies depending on clinical status.

Role of Central Venous and Intra-abdominal Pressure

Increased intra-abdominal pressure (IAP) can result in intra-abdominal hypertension (IAH) and abdominal compartment syndrome (ACS) in severe cases. IAH is defined as an unrelenting increased IAP of greater than or equal to 12 mm Hg, and IAP greater than 20 mm Hg defines ACS.[28] IAP increases are traditionally seen and discussed in the context of surgical complications but are now increasingly recognized as an important pathophysiologic contribution to the CRS.

ADHF results in volume overload and increased central venous pressure (CVP). To maintain blood flow through the vascular system an adequate pressure gradient is required across the capillary network. Increased venous pressures attenuate the gradient for forward blood flow across the renal vasculature, resulting in sluggish flow and causing congestion, glomerular dysfunction, and a decrease in urine output. Various studies have shown that increased IAP results in reduced GFR and renal plasma flow[29,30] and that an increased CVP is significantly associated with decreased kidney function.

In a study of 40 patients with ADHF, 60% of patients had increased IAP. Patients with increased IAP ($\geq$8 mm Hg) at baseline had higher serum creatinine levels compared with those with normal IAP (2.3 $\pm$ 1.0 mg/dL vs 1.5 $\pm$ 0.8 mg/dL; $P =$ .009, respectively). Intensive medical therapy resulted in significant reduction in right-sided and left-sided filling pressures and an improvement in cardiac index (CI); these hemodynamic improvements did not correlate with improvements in renal function or IAP. However, changes in IAP did correlate with changes in renal function. This disconnect between hemodynamics and IAP likely explains why a subset of patients have deterioration in renal function despite improvement in hemodynamics because they have a persistent increase in IAP at follow-up.[31]

Although increased IAP and IAH have an important role in renal dysfunction, increases in CVP have also been shown to closely correlate with renal function. A retrospective study conducted on patients who underwent right heart catheterization showed that an increased CVP (>6 mm Hg) was associated with impaired renal function as well as being a strong and independent predictor of all-cause mortality.[32] Similarly, another study of 145 patients with ADHF found that CVPs were higher in persons who developed WRF compared with those who did not (18 $\pm$ 7 mm Hg vs 12 $\pm$ 6 mm Hg; P<.001).[33] In addition, the mean baseline CI was higher in subjects who developed WRF, suggesting that CVP may be more closely associated with eGFR than CI. Furthermore, a study of 196 patients with HF showed that tricuspid regurgitation was independently associated with lower GFR.[34] Significant tricuspid regurgitation can impair venous return and reflux blood into the renal-hepatic system.

Role of Cardiac Output and Cardiac Index

Initially, much of the progressive decline in renal function observed with HF was thought to be secondary to poor renal perfusion from a reduced cardiac output. The hypothesized pathophysiology being that inadequate renal blood flow or perfusion pressure prompts renin release by the juxtaglomerular cells of the afferent arterioles because of a low-flow state in the ascending limb of the

Table 2
Summary of various mechanisms of cardiorenal syndrome

Mechanism	Mediator	End-organ Outcome	
		Heart	Kidney
• Increased central venous and intra-abdominal pressures	• Increased salt/water retention • Activation of RAAS/SNS	• Acute/chronic HF • Adverse remodeling of heart and lungs	• Renal venous congestion • Reduced GFR
• Reduced cardiac output and cardiac index	• Peripheral vasodilation/reduced vascular resistance • Reduced perfusion pressure	• Activation of RAAS/SNS detrimental to heart • Cardiac ischemia from reduced perfusion	• Reduced renal perfusion • Renal ischemia

• Neurohormonal dysregulation
  ○ RAAS activation
  ○ SNS activation
  ○ Adenosine/AVP
	• Impaired baroreceptor reflexes
	• Increased renin secretion
	• Increased Ang II secretion
	• Increased aldosterone secretion
	• Increased ET-1 expression
	• Oxidative stress
		• Myocyte hypertrophy, left ventricular dysfunction
		• Proinflammation, profibrotic effect
		• Hypertension
			• Arteriolar vasoconstriction
			• Reduced GFR
			• Enhanced reabsorption of sodium/water
			• Proinflammation, profibrotic effect

• Oxidative stress	• Increased reactive oxygen species formation • Ang II–enhanced NADPH-oxidase activity • Uremic toxin–mediated cytokine release	• Left ventricular hypertrophy • Accelerated atherosclerosis • Endothelial dysfunction • Inflammation • Fibrosis	• Endothelial dysfunction • Accelerated atherosclerosis • Inflammation • Interstitial fibrosis
• Inflammatory mediators	• TNF-α • TWEAK • Members of IL-1 family • IL-6 • CRP	• Atherosclerosis • Inflammation • Left ventricular dysfunction • Cardiac hypertrophy • Myocardial cell death • Fibrosis	• Inflammation • Fibrosis • Atherosclerosis • Glomerular damage by mesangial cell apoptosis
• Renal failure–disturbances	• PBUTs (indoxyl sulfate, p-cresyl sulfate) • Chronic inflammatory cytokines • Oxidative stress • FGF-23 • Calcium/phosphate-mediated inflammation • Anemia	• Endothelial dysfunction • Atherosclerosis • Left ventricular dysfunction • Cardiac hypertrophy	• Atherosclerosis • Inflammation • Increased interstitial and perivascular fibrosis

Abbreviations: Ang II, angiotensin II; AVP, arginine vasopressin; CRP, C-reactive protein; ET-1, endothelin-1; FGF-23, fibroblast growth factor-23; GFR, glomerular filtration rate; IL, interleukin; PBUTs, protein-bound uremic toxins; RAAS, renin-angiotensin-aldosterone system; SNS, sympathetic nervous system; TNF-α, tumor necrosis factor alpha; TWEAK, tumor necrosis factor alpha–related weak inducer of apoptosis.

loop of Henle and the pressure-sensing baroreceptors. This release leads to:

- The retention of sodium
- Increased vascular congestion

- Further worsening of renal function caused by renal afferent arteriolar vasoconstriction

In an animal study, an impaired response to an acute sodium load in rats with left ventricular dysfunction secondary to healed myocardial infarction showed a model of circulatory impairment.[35] In theory, by augmenting contractility, heart rate, and CI, inotropes can lead to a short-term improvement in urine output, mental status, and other clinical indicators of organ perfusion. However, investigations suggest that this concept is limited and management of patients with CRS based solely on the low-flow theory does not lead to improved outcomes. This suggestion is supported by findings from Evaluation Study of Congestive Heart Failure and Pulmonary Artery Catheterization Effectiveness (ESCAPE) study, a trial evaluating hemodynamically guided management of ADHF (using a pulmonary artery catheter) versus usual clinical care.[36] Among the 433 individuals admitted with ADHF, the investigators found no correlation between baseline renal function and CI. Furthermore, improvement in CI did not result in improved renal function, prevention of death, or prevention of rehospitalization. An important caveat of the ESCAPE trial was that patients were excluded if in cardiogenic shock or investigators thought that invasive hemodynamic monitoring was clinically indicated.

Counter to these findings, a more recent study of patients with acute cardiogenic shock did find an association between decreased CI and AKI.[37] This population was excluded from the ESCAPE trial, and these results suggest that, in patients with an acute severe decline in cardiac output or a markedly depressed cardiac output, a low-forward-flow pathophysiologic state contributes to CRS. Despite this theory of low forward flow, treatment with inotropic agents in various groups of patients with HF and AKI did not change the clinical outcomes and further endorses the fact that CRS pathophysiology and management is far more complicated than previously thought.[38,39] Thus, in the acute setting, the influence of CI is variable and may contribute to the most severe forms of ADHF but likely does not play a significant role in most patients.

Although these studies investigated ADHF, data are more limited in congestive HF (CHF). One study evaluated a large cohort of patients undergoing right heart catheterization without a clear discrimination of acuity or stability of HF status. CI correlated with renal function but was not the sole contributing hemodynamic process.[32] As discussed earlier, CVP is another dominant hemodynamic factor influencing renal function.

Role of Neurohormonal Dysregulation

The renin-angiotensin-aldosterone system (RAAS) plays an important role in the progression of kidney damage and worsening of HF.[40] In patients with HF, neurohormonal mechanisms are activated to restore tissue perfusion. In addition, in HF overactivity of the sympathetic nervous system (SNS) caused by impaired baroreceptor reflexes results in increased renin release from the juxtamedullary cells of the kidneys.[41] Renin synthesis is also influenced by the hydrostatic pressure sensed at glomerular afferent arterioles, and the reduced quantity of chloride delivered to the macula densa.[42] An increase in renin level leads to increased production of angiotensin II (Ang II), which has multiple maladaptive systemic effects on the heart, vasculature, and kidneys. In the kidneys, Ang II causes renal efferent arteriolar vasoconstriction and an increased fraction of renal plasma flow filtered across the glomerulus, which results in an increased peritubular oncotic pressure and reduced hydrostatic pressure causing enhanced reabsorption of sodium in the proximal tubules. Ang II has a direct stimulating effect on proximal tubule sodium bicarbonate cotransporters and apical sodium hydrogen exchangers, through which solute is proximally reabsorbed independent of the GFR.[43] Ang II also promotes the aldosterone-mediated reabsorption of sodium in the distal tubules[42] and increases the expression of endothelin-1 (ET-1) in the kidney.[44] ET-1 is a potent vasoconstrictor, a proinflammatory and profibrotic peptide, and leads to pathologic changes resulting in kidney injury.[45]

Ang II type 1 (AT_1) receptors are also found in the heart. In animal models, stimulation of AT_1 receptors results in cardiac myocyte hypertrophy through paracrine release of transforming growth factor-β_1 and ET-1 from the cardiac fibroblast.[46] Ang II causes vascular smooth muscle contraction via the AT_1 receptors. Furthermore, Ang II mediates the oxidative stress via reactive oxygen species (ROS) formation in the heart and kidney tissue leading to inflammation and hypertension.[47] In patients with HF, left ventricular dysfunction causes activation of SNS in an effort to maintain the perfusion through mechanisms such as increased contractility, lusitropy, and systemic vasoconstriction.[48]

Adenosine is released in response to an increased sodium load in the distal tubule and via adenosine type 1 receptors in the proximal tubule and afferent arterioles; it mediates constriction of afferent arterioles and reduction of renal blood flow and GFR. In addition, activation of adenosine type 2 receptors induces the release of renin and enhances sodium reabsorption at the proximal tubule and reduces diuresis.[49] Efficacy of adenosine type 1 receptor antagonist in CRS is controversial. The results of the PROTECT (A Placebo-controlled Randomized Study of the

Selective A1 Adenosine Receptor Antagonist Rolofylline for Patients Hospitalized with ADHF to Assess Treatment Effect on Congestion and Renal Function) trial showed that the rolofylline group did not meet the primary (dyspnea improvement) or secondary (death, cardiovascular or renal rehospitalization, or persistent renal impairment) outcomes. Thus, further clinical studies are needed to determine the utility of adenosine A1 receptor antagonist in the CRS population.[50]

Arginine vasopressin (AVP) is a nonapeptide synthesized in the hypothalamus, stimulated in response to serum osmolality. It has effects on glomerular hemodynamics, arterial blood pressure, and nonhemodynamic renal mechanisms. Patients with ADHF often have an activation of AVP release. AVP causes water retention via vasopressin V2 (V2) receptors in the collecting duct. Studies have shown that increased AVP levels contribute to the progression of CKD.[51,52] The renal hemodynamic effects of AVP may be caused by its effects on the RAAS. AVP could potentially stimulate renin secretion directly via activation of V2 receptors or indirectly through reduction in sodium concentration at the macula densa.[51] Plasma AVP level has been found to be increased in patients with left ventricular dysfunction without overt clinical HF and has been associated with poor outcomes.[53,54]

Role of Oxidative Stress

Oxidative stress is defined as an imbalance between oxidants and antioxidants resulting in excessive accumulation of the former leading to cellular injury.[55] ROS are generated as by-products of cellular metabolism, primarily in the mitochondria.[56] Oxidative stress ensues when formation of ROS surpasses the body's antioxidative processing ability, resulting in the accumulation of ROS leading to cellular damage, endothelial dysfunction, and progression of atherosclerosis.

Oxidative stress in the setting of CRS can be triggered by ischemic injury, venous congestion (which causes circumferential wall stress in the endothelial cell membrane), and inflammation.[57,58] Most of the adenosine triphosphate (ATP) is produced from fatty acid oxidation in the heart, but in the setting of HF there is a shift from fatty acid oxidation to glycolysis in myocytes, leading to myocardial ATP production decreasing by 30% to 40%. The energy deficiency is compensated by glycolysis but it is insufficient to meet the energy needs in HF, leading to low threshold for hypoxemia, apoptosis, and cell death. Furthermore, because of reduced mitochondrial oxidative metabolism of fatty acid oxidation, there is

accumulation of free fatty acids in myocytes, leading to lipotoxicity.[59] In a study, patients admitted with ADHF who subsequently developed AKI were studied for markers of oxidative stress (interleukin [IL]-6, myeloperoxidase, nitric oxide, copper/zinc superoxide dismutase, and endogenous peroxidase). Results showed significantly heightened presence of dual oxidative stress markers in patients who developed CRS type 1.[60]

In addition to the deleterious effects of volume expansion and hemodynamics, RAAS and SNS activation also play an important role in amplifying the oxidative stress in patients with HF and CKD. Ang II has a deleterious effect by activating NADPH-oxidase–promoting oxidative injury by producing ROS causing mitochondrial dysfunction.[61] The enhanced NADPH-oxidase activity has been shown in endothelial cells, renal tubular cells, and cardiac myocytes.[62–64]

Patients with advance CKD and end-stage renal disease (ESRD) have some factors, such as uremic toxins and dialysate solutions used in renal replacement therapy, that could lead to increased synthesis and release of proinflammatory cytokines, oxidative stress, immune system dysregulation leading to carotid artery intima-media thickness (marker of early stage of atherosclerosis), and left ventricular hypertrophy.[65,66] Patients with ESRD have higher cardiovascular morbidity and mortality that could not be explained by classic cardiac risk factors; thus, oxidative stress, endothelial dysfunction, and hyperhomocysteinemia might be playing an additive role in these patients.[67]

Role of Inflammatory Mediators

Both CKD and HF are states of heightened chronic inflammation, resulting in the generation of proinflammatory biomarkers that play a crucial role in tissue damage to both organs leading to cell death and fibrosis. Important triggers that initiate and propagate the inflammatory cascade include the activation of SNS and RAAS, venous congestion, ischemia, and oxidative stress. Proinflammatory cytokines such as tumor necrosis factor alpha (TNF-α) and TNF-α–related weak inducer of apoptosis (TWEAK), members of the IL-1 family, and IL-6 have been associated with HF as well as CKD. In kidneys, TNF-α and IL-6 promote accumulation of inflammatory cells in the interstitium by increasing expression of monocyte chemoattractant proteins. TNF-α also results in glomerular damage by mesangial cell apoptosis.[68] Some of these biomarkers are prognostic for all-cause mortality in patients with HF, such as soluble ST2, which is a member of the IL-1 family.[69,70]

Similarly, in CKD, IL-6 correlates well with progression of disease and also predicts the mortality.[71] It has also been shown that levels of these proinflammatory markers are higher in persons with CKD[72] and those on dialysis.[73]

C-reactive protein (CRP), an acute phase reactant, has been shown to contribute to the pathogenesis of atherosclerosis through a variety of mechanisms. CRP activates the complement system and is widely distributed in early atherosclerotic lesions.[74,75] CRP is a potent stimulator of tissue factor production (a potent procoagulant) by monocytes, and this effect is further augmented in the presence of inflammatory mediators.[76] In a study of 4269 individuals hospitalized with ADHF, patients with CRP in the fourth quartile ($\geq$9.6 mg/L) were independently associated with higher all-cause mortality (adjusted hazard ratio, 1.68) within 120 days after discharge.[77] In hemodialysis patients, high CRP levels predict left ventricular dysfunction, cardiac hypertrophy, and mortality.[78,79] These inflammatory proteins are not simply inert markers of disease activity but play an active and complex role in the pathophysiology of CRS.

Role of Renal Failure–associated Disturbances

Protein-bound uremic toxins (PBUTs) are currently an emerging area of interest because of their potential association with cardiovascular disease.[80,81] Indoxyl sulfate (IS) and p-cresyl sulfate (PCS) are the two most extensively studied PBUTs that have shown a role in the pathogenesis and progression of CRS. In normal kidneys, both are cleared through tubular secretion. Experimental studies have shown a detrimental effect of IS and PCS through alteration of oxidative stress, endothelial dysfunction, and atherosclerosis. Both have been associated with nephrotoxicity, decreased endothelial proliferation, and impaired wound repair, suggesting their role in the progression of CKD.[82-85] A study using a nephrectomy CKD mouse model revealed effects of PCS on cardiac cells, including increased apoptosis, increased interstitial and perivascular fibrosis, and a reduction in left ventricular diastolic function. Oxidative stress was implicated in PCS-induced changes in the heart muscle.[86] Furthermore, IS also augments oxidative stress in kidney and heart, leading to cardiorenal fibrosis.[87-89] A study of 139 patients with CKD showed that IS was a powerful predictor of overall and cardiovascular mortality after adjusting for confounders.[90] Although there has been evidence suggesting a negative effect of PBUTs on heart, kidney, and vascular cells, further research is needed to better understand the role of PBUTs in the pathophysiology of CRS.

Fibroblast growth factor-23 (FGF23), a hormone produced in the bone that controls phosphate and vitamin D metabolism by the kidney, is a strong predictor of adverse cardiovascular outcomes in patients with CKD and ESRD. Increased FGF-23 level has been associated with left ventricular hypertrophy and mortality in patients with advanced CKD.[91] Although it has been suggested that FGF23 may induce myocardial hypertrophy through a direct effect on cardiac myocytes, this remains debated because of the absence of alpha-klotho receptors (which mediate FGF23 action) in the heart. Other data also suggest that FGF23 may directly depress myocardial contractility and ventricular relaxation, cause hypertrophy, and increase risk of arrhythmias by altering calcium trafficking.[92,93]

Role of Anemia

Anemia is common in patients with advanced CKD and HF, and most of these patients have anemia of chronic disease. The prevalence of anemia in CRS has been reported to vary from 5% to 55%, with anemia reported to be an independent predictor of mortality.[94-96] In the OPTIMIZE-HF (Organized Program to Initiate Lifesaving Treatment in Hospitalized Patients With Heart Failure) registry with more than 48,000 patients, 51.2% had mild anemia (hemoglobin level <12.1 g/dL) and 25% were moderately to severely anemic (hemoglobin levels of 5–10.7 g/dL).[97]

In a multicenter survey of 5222 patients with CKD, 47.7% were found to be anemic (hemoglobin level $\leq$12 g/dL).[98]

In patients with CKD, anemia is associated with:

- Cognitive impairment
- Poor quality of life
- Progression of kidney disease
- Cardiovascular comorbidities
- Higher mortality[99]

There are several ways anemia contributes to the pathophysiology of CRS. Lack of oxygen supply to a heart that is already under stress or kidney that is already damaged may cause ischemic insults that can result in progressive cell death in both the organs. Red blood cells contain many antioxidants, and therefore anemia may result in increased oxidative stress.[100] Anemia can cause tissue ischemia and peripheral vasodilation, which leads to activation of SNS, RAAS, as well as release of antidiuretic hormone, resulting in vasoconstriction, salt and water retention, and chronic renal venous congestion that leads to progressive nephron loss and interstitial fibrosis. Chronic anemic state also results in left ventricular hypertrophy and myocardial cell death from ischemia and necrosis.[101,102]

Although correction of anemia in patients with CHF with erythropoiesis-stimulating agents results in improved outcomes (reduced hospitalization; improved New York Heart Association class, 6-minute walk test, and quality of life) but normalization of the hemoglobin levels may not result in favorable outcomes. Trials targeting higher hemoglobin levels ($\geq$13 g/dL) were surprisingly associated with higher rate of adverse events.[103,104] The Trial to Reduce Cardiovascular Events with Aranesp Therapy (TREAT) was a randomized, double-blind, placebo-controlled study with more than 4000 patients.[105] The use of darbepoetin alfa in patients with diabetes, CKD, and moderate anemia who were not undergoing dialysis to achieve a hemoglobin level of approximately 13 g/dL did not reduce the risk of death, cardiovascular event, or renal event. There was an increased risk of fatal or nonfatal stroke in patients assigned to the darbepoetin alfa group. The RED-HF (Reduction of Events by Darbepoetin Alfa in Heart Failure) was a randomized, double-blind trial with 2278 patients with systolic heart failure and mild to moderate anemia (hemoglobin level, 9.0–12.0 g/dL).[106] Patients were randomized to either darbepoetin alfa (to achieve a hemoglobin target of 13 g/dL) or placebo. There was no difference in the primary outcome (death from any cause or hospitalization for worsening HF).

Anemia plays an important role in the pathophysiology of CRS, and management of anemia is complex, especially in patients with CKD and CHF. The main unanswered question is the range of hemoglobin levels to target in this population; targets based on CKD guidelines (10–12 g/dL) or higher (12–13 g/dL) but less than 13 g/dL (because trials with hemoglobin level of 13 g/dL or greater were associated with negative outcomes) is still unknown.

Pathogenesis of Type 5 Cardiorenal Syndrome

Type 5 CRS (CRS-5) occurs when an overwhelming systemic disease process results in damage to heart and kidney simultaneously (**Fig. 4**). Based on pathophysiology and severity of the disease process, CRS-5 has been classified into 4 stages: hyperacute, acute, subacute, and chronic. Systemic diseases that can result in CRS-5 are sepsis, connective tissue disorders such as lupus, sarcoidosis, amyloidosis, and

Cardiorenal syndrome type 5

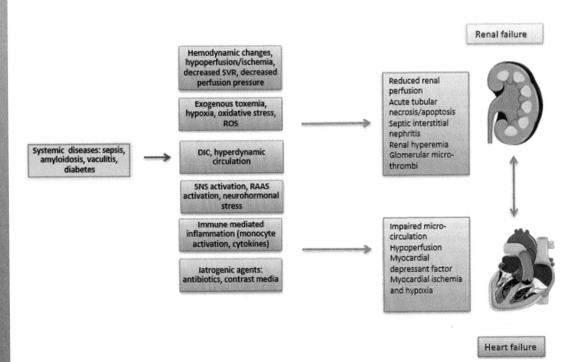

Fig. 4. Pathophysiologic interactions in cardiorenal syndrome (type 5). DIC, disseminated intravascular coagulation; SVR, systemic vascular resistance.

cirrhosis. Injury to the kidney and heart is often mediated by proinflammatory cytokines, complement factors, and RAAS activation, which are often the common end pathway for other forms of CRS. For instance, in sepsis, increased renal vascular resistance and early increase in proinflammatory cytokines (IL-6) and oxidative stress can lead to organ damage.[107,108] Sepsis also results in autonomic nervous system dysfunction and activation of RAAS. The plethora of effects of sepsis on the function of various organs, including heart and kidney, makes it difficult to differentiate between the effects of sepsis and the effect of interorgan crosstalk. Moreover, management of sepsis can contribute to the development of CRS-5. Fluid resuscitation can result in tissue edema and IAH, increased venous congestion, and reduced renal perfusion. Iodinated contrast agents and certain drugs can result in myocardial depression and nephrotoxicity, resulting in development and/or worsening of CRS-5. In chronic inflammatory and autoimmune disease processes, the concomitant damage to both the organs and ongoing crosstalk between the heart and kidney leads to a similar pathophysiologic mechanism as discussed in other types of CRS.[109]

FUTURE DIRECTIONS

Despite an improved understanding of the different pathophysiologic processes involved in the development of CRS, therapies intended to improve outcomes in this population have only met with minimal success. One possibility for this may be the inability to accurately diagnose AKI using conventional biomarkers such as creatinine. Whether the incorporation of more novel filtration markers, such as cystatin C, beta-2 microglobulin, and beta trace protein, will provide better estimates of kidney function needs to be evaluated further in the setting of HF. Further, based on emerging evidence, there is a need to incorporate more sensitive, and perhaps specific, tubular markers of injury, inflammation, and repair into the renal end points of HF clinical trials.[110]

SUMMARY

The pathophysiology of the various types of CRS is complex and challenging. Given the increasing burden of the disease, adverse clinical outcomes, and high impact on mortality, early diagnosis of the syndrome is crucial. To improve the survival and morbidity associated with the disease, better understanding of various aspects of pathophysiology is needed to better manage these patients. CRS-5 is a complex and challenging condition to diagnose because the timing and sequence of dysfunction of heart and kidney are dictated by the underlying cause and nature of condition.

REFERENCES

1. Cardio-renal connections in heart failure and cardiovascular disease | National Heart, Lung, and Blood Institute (NHLBI). Available at: https://www.nhlbi.nih.gov/events/2004/cardio-renal-connections-heart-failure-and-cardiovascular-disease. Accessed January 15, 2019.
2. House AA, Anand I, Bellomo R, et al. Definition and classification of cardio-renal syndromes: workgroup statements from the 7th ADQI consensus conference. Nephrol Dial Transplant 2010;25(5): 1416–20.
3. Ronco C, McCullough P, Anker SD, et al. Cardiorenal syndromes: report from the consensus conference of the acute dialysis quality initiative. Eur Heart J 2009;31(6):703–11.
4. Berl T, Henrich W. Kidney-heart interactions: epidemiology, pathogenesis, and treatment. Clin J Am Soc Nephrol 2006;1(1):8–18.
5. Ronco C, House AA, Haapio M. Cardiorenal syndrome: refining the definition of a complex symbiosis gone wrong. Intensive Care Med 2008; 34(5):957.
6. Health, United States. With special feature on mortality, 87, 2017. Available at: https://www.cdc.gov/nchs/data/hus/hus17.pdf.
7. Damman K, Tang WHW, Testani JM, et al. Terminology and definition of changes renal function in heart failure. Eur Heart J 2014;35(48):3413–6.
8. Khwaja A. KDIGO clinical practice guidelines for acute kidney injury. Nephron Clin Pract 2012; 120(4):c179–84.
9. Testani JM, McCauley BD, Chen J, et al. Worsening renal function defined as an absolute increase in serum creatinine is a biased metric for the study of cardio-renal interactions. Cardiology 2010; 116(3):206–12.
10. Ambrosy AP, Pang PS, Khan S, et al. Clinical course and predictive value of congestion during hospitalization in patients admitted for worsening signs and symptoms of heart failure with reduced ejection fraction: findings from the EVEREST trial. Eur Heart J 2013;34(11):835–43.
11. Lala A, McNulty SE, Mentz RJ, et al. Relief and recurrence of congestion during and after hospitalization for acute heart failure: insights from diuretic optimization strategy evaluation in acute decompensated heart failure (DOSE-AHF) and cardiorenal rescue study in acute decompensated heart failure (CARESS-HF). Circ Heart Fail 2015;8(4):741–8.

12. Fonarow GC, Stough WG, Abraham WT, et al. Characteristics, treatments, and outcomes of patients with preserved systolic function hospitalized for heart failure: a report from the OPTIMIZE-HF registry. J Am Coll Cardiol 2007;50(8):768–77.

13. Levin A, Stevens PE, Bilous RW, et al. Kidney Disease: improving Global Outcomes (KDIGO) CKD Work Group. KDIGO 2012 clinical practice guideline for the evaluation and management of chronic kidney disease. Kidney Int Suppl 2013;3(1):1–150.

14. Jackson CE, Solomon SD, Gerstein HC, et al. Albuminuria in chronic heart failure: prevalence and prognostic importance. Lancet 2009;374(9689): 543–50.

15. Ninomiya T, Perkovic V, de Galan BE, et al. Albuminuria and kidney function independently predict cardiovascular and renal outcomes in diabetes. J Am Soc Nephrol 2009;20(8):1813–21.

16. Astor BC, Hallan SI, Miller ER, et al. Glomerular filtration rate, albuminuria, and risk of cardiovascular and all-cause mortality in the US population. Am J Epidemiol 2008;167(10):1226–34.

17. Heywood JT, Fonarow GC, Costanzo MR, et al. High prevalence of renal dysfunction and its impact on outcome in 118,465 patients hospitalized with acute decompensated heart failure: a report from the ADHERE database. J Card Fail 2007;13(6):422–30.

18. Damman K, Valente MAE, Voors AA, et al. Renal impairment, worsening renal function, and outcome in patients with heart failure: an updated meta-analysis. Eur Heart J 2014;35(7):455–69.

19. Metra M, Davison B, Bettari L, et al. Is worsening renal function an ominous prognostic sign in patients with acute heart failure? The role of congestion and its interaction with renal function. Circ Heart Fail 2012;5(1):54–62.

20. Khan NA, Ma I, Thompson CR, et al. Kidney function and mortality among patients with left ventricular systolic dysfunction. J Am Soc Nephrol 2006; 17(1):244–53.

21. Testani JM, Kimmel SE, Dries DL, et al. Prognostic importance of early worsening renal function following initiation of angiotensin converting enzyme inhibitor therapy in patients with cardiac dysfunction. Circ Heart Fail 2011;4(6):685–91.

22. Testani JM, McCauley BD, Chen J, et al. Clinical characteristics and outcomes of patients with improvement in renal function during the treatment of decompensated heart failure. J Card Fail 2011; 17(12):993–1000.

23. Brisco MA, Zile MR, Hanberg JS, et al. Relevance of changes in serum creatinine during a heart failure trial of decongestive strategies: insights from the DOSE trial. J Card Fail 2016;22(10):753–60.

24. McCullough PA, Kellum JA, Haase M, et al. Pathophysiology of the cardiorenal syndromes: executive summary from the eleventh consensus conference of the Acute Dialysis Quality Initiative (ADQI). Contrib Nephrol 2013;182:82–98.

25. Cruz DN, Schmidt-Ott KM, Vescovo G, et al. Pathophysiology of cardiorenal syndrome type 2 in stable chronic heart failure: workgroup statements from the eleventh consensus conference of the Acute Dialysis Quality Initiative (ADQI). Contrib Nephrol 2013;182:117–36.

26. Ahmad T, Jackson K, Rao Veena S, et al. Worsening renal function in patients with acute heart failure undergoing aggressive diuresis is not associated with tubular injury. Circulation 2018;137(19): 2016–28.

27. Bart BA, Goldsmith SR, Lee KL, et al. Ultrafiltration in decompensated heart failure with cardiorenal syndrome. N Engl J Med 2012;367(24):2296–304.

28. Malbrain ML, Cheatham ML, Kirkpatrick A, et al. Results from the international conference of experts on intra-abdominal hypertension and abdominal compartment syndrome. I. Definitions. Intensive Care Med 2006;32(11):1722–32.

29. Bradley SE, Bradley GP. The effect of increased intra-abdominal pressure on renal function in man 1. J Clin Invest 1947;26(5):1010–22.

30. Dalfino L, Tullo L, Donadio I, et al. Intra-abdominal hypertension and acute renal failure in critically ill patients. Intensive Care Med 2008;34(4):707–13.

31. Mullens W, Abrahams Z, Skouri HN, et al. Elevated intra-abdominal pressure in acute decompensated heart failure: a potential contributor to worsening renal function? J Am Coll Cardiol 2008;51(3): 300–6.

32. Damman K, van Deursen VM, Navis G, et al. Increased central venous pressure is associated with impaired renal function and mortality in a broad spectrum of patients with cardiovascular disease. J Am Coll Cardiol 2009;53(7):582–8.

33. Mullens W, Abrahams Z, Francis GS, et al. Importance of venous congestion for worsening of renal function in advanced decompensated heart failure. J Am Coll Cardiol 2009;53(7):589–96.

34. Maeder MT, Holst DP, Kaye DM. Tricuspid regurgitation contributes to renal dysfunction in patients with heart failure. J Card Fail 2008;14(10):824–30.

35. Hostetter TH, Pfeffer JM, Pfeffer MA, et al. Cardiorenal hemodynamics and sodium excretion in rats with myocardial infarction. Am J Physiol 1983;245(1):H98–103.

36. Binanay C, Califf RM, Hasselblad V, et al. Evaluation study of congestive heart failure and pulmonary artery catheterization effectiveness: the ESCAPE trial. JAMA 2005;294(13):1625–33.

37. Tarvasmäki T, Haapio M, Mebazaa A, et al. Acute kidney injury in cardiogenic shock: definitions, incidence, haemodynamic alterations, and mortality. Eur J Heart Fail 2018;20(3):572–81.

38. Bellomo R, Chapman M, Finfer S, et al. Low-dose dopamine in patients with early renal dysfunction: a placebo-controlled randomised trial. Australian and New Zealand Intensive Care Society (ANZICS) Clinical Trials Group. Lancet 2000;356(9248): 2139–43.

39. Lauschke A, Teichgräber UKM, Frei U, et al. 'Low-dose' dopamine worsens renal perfusion in patients with acute renal failure. Kidney Int 2006; 69(9):1669–74.

40. Ferrario CM, Strawn WB. Role of the renin-angiotensin-aldosterone system and proinflammatory mediators in cardiovascular disease. Am J Cardiol 2006;98(1):121–8.

41. Kopp UC. Neural control of renin secretion rate. Morgan & Claypool Life Sciences; 2011. Available at: https://www.ncbi.nlm.nih.gov/books/NBK57240/. Accessed January 3, 2019.

42. Harrison-Bernard LM. The renal renin-angiotensin system. Adv Physiol Educ 2009;33(4):270–4.

43. Johnson MD, Malvin RL. Stimulation of renal sodium reabsorption by angiotensin II. Am J Physiol 1977;232(4):F298–306.

44. Barton M, Shaw S, d'uscio LV, et al. Angiotensin II increases vascular and renal endothelin-1 and functional endothelin converting enzyme activity in vivo: role of ETA receptors for endothelin regulation. Biochem Biophys Res Commun 1997;238(3): 861–5.

45. Neuhofer W, Pittrow D. Role of endothelin and endothelin receptor antagonists in renal disease. Eur J Clin Invest 2006;36(s3):78–88.

46. Gray MO, Long CS, Kalinyak JE, et al. Angiotensin II stimulates cardiac myocyte hypertrophy via paracrine release of TGF-β1 and endothelin-1 from fibroblasts. Cardiovasc Res 1998;40(2): 352–63.

47. Hitomi H, Kiyomoto H, Nishiyama A. Angiotensin II and oxidative stress. Curr Opin Cardiol 2007;22(4): 311–5.

48. Triposkiadis F, Karayannis G, Giamouzis G, et al. The sympathetic nervous system in heart failure: physiology, pathophysiology, and clinical implications. J Am Coll Cardiol 2009; 54(19):1747–62.

49. Funaya H, Kitakaze M, Node K, et al. Plasma adenosine levels increase in patients with chronic heart failure. Circulation 1997;95(6):1363–5.

50. Massie BM, O'Connor CM, Metra M, et al. Rolofylline, an adenosine A1–Receptor antagonist, in acute heart failure. N Engl J Med 2010;363(15): 1419–28.

51. Bardoux P, Martin H, Ahloulay M, et al. Vasopressin contributes to hyperfiltration, albuminuria, and renal hypertrophy in diabetes mellitus: study in vasopressin-deficient Brattleboro rats. Proc Natl Acad Sci U S A 1999;96(18):10397–402.

52. Torres VE. Vasopressin in chronic kidney disease, an elephant in the room? Kidney Int 2009;76(9): 925–8.

53. Francis GS, Benedict C, Johnstone DE, et al. Comparison of neuroendocrine activation in patients with left ventricular dysfunction with and without congestive heart failure. A substudy of the Studies of Left Ventricular Dysfunction (SOLVD). Circulation 1990;82(5):1724–9.

54. Rouleau JL, Packer M, Moyé L, et al. Prognostic value of neurohumoral activation in patients with an acute myocardial infarction: effect of captopril. J Am Coll Cardiol 1994;24(3):583–91.

55. Sies H. Oxidative stress: oxidants and antioxidants. Exp Physiol 1997;82(2):291–5.

56. Thannickal VJ, Fanburg BL. Reactive oxygen species in cell signaling. Am J Physiol Lung Cell Mol Physiol 2000;279(6):L1005–28.

57. Colombo PC, Doran AC, Onat D, et al. Venous congestion, endothelial and neurohormonal activation in acute decompensated heart failure: cause or effect? Curr Heart Fail Rep 2015;12(3):215–22.

58. Rubattu S, Mennuni S, Testa M, et al. Pathogenesis of chronic cardiorenal syndrome: is there a role for oxidative stress? Int J Mol Sci 2013;14(11): 23011–32.

59. Katz AM, Konstam MA. Heart failure: pathophysiology, molecular biology, and clinical management. Lippincott Williams & Wilkins; 2012.

60. Virzì GM, Clementi A, de Cal M, et al. Oxidative stress: dual pathway induction in cardiorenal syndrome type 1 pathogenesis. Oxid Med Cell Longev 2015;2015. https://doi.org/10.1155/2015/391790.

61. Kimura S, Zhang G, Nishiyama A, et al. Role of NAD(P)H oxidase- and mitochondria-derived reactive oxygen species in cardioprotection of ischemic reperfusion injury by angiotensin II. Hypertension 2005;45(5):860–6.

62. Nakagami H, Takemoto M, Liao JK. NADPH oxidase-derived superoxide anion mediates angiotensin II-induced cardiac hypertrophy. J Mol Cell Cardiol 2003;35(7):851–9.

63. Chabrashvili T, Kitiyakara C, Blau J, et al. Effects of ANG II type 1 and 2 receptors on oxidative stress, renal NADPH oxidase, and SOD expression. Am J Physiol Regul Integr Comp Physiol 2003;285(1): R117–24.

64. Ushio-Fukai M, Zafari AM, Fukui T, et al. P22phox is a critical component of the superoxide-generating NADH/NADPH oxidase system and regulates angiotensin II-induced hypertrophy in vascular smooth muscle cells. J Biol Chem 1996;271(38): 23317–21.

65. Granata S, Zaza G, Simone S, et al. Mitochondrial dysregulation and oxidative stress in patients with chronic kidney disease. BMC Genomics 2009;10: 388.

66. Modaresi A, Nafar M, Sahraei Z. Oxidative stress in chronic kidney disease 2015;9(3):15.

67. Becker BN, Himmelfarb J, Henrich WL, et al. Re-assessing the cardiac risk profile in chronic hemodialysis patients: a hypothesis on the role of oxidant stress and other non-traditional cardiac risk factors. J Am Soc Nephrol 1997;8(3):475–86. Available at: https://jasn.asnjournals.org/content/8/3/475. Accessed January 21, 2019.

68. Radeke HH, Meier B, Topley N, et al. Interleukin 1-alpha and tumor necrosis factor-alpha induce oxygen radical production in mesangial cells. Kidney Int 1990;37(2):767–75.

69. Tsutamoto T, Hisanaga T, Wada A, et al. Interleukin-6 spillover in the peripheral circulation increases with the severity of heart failure, and the high plasma level of interleukin-6 is an important prognostic predictor in patients with congestive heart failure. J Am Coll Cardiol 1998;31(2):391–8.

70. Wettersten N, Maisel AS. Biomarkers for heart failure: an update for practitioners of internal medicine. Am J Med 2016;129(6):560–7.

71. Barreto DV, Barreto FC, Liabeuf S, et al. Plasma interleukin-6 is independently associated with mortality in both hemodialysis and pre-dialysis patients with chronic kidney disease. Kidney Int 2010;77(6):550–6.

72. Stenvinkel P, Ketteler M, Johnson RJ, et al. IL-10, IL-6, and TNF-alpha: central factors in the altered cytokine network of uremia–the good, the bad, and the ugly. Kidney Int 2005;67(4):1216–33.

73. Pereira BJ, Shapiro L, King AJ, et al. Plasma levels of IL-1 beta, TNF alpha and their specific inhibitors in undialyzed chronic renal failure, CAPD and hemodialysis patients. Kidney Int 1994;45(3):890–6.

74. Torzewski J, Torzewski M, Bowyer DE, et al. C-reactive protein frequently colocalizes with the terminal complement complex in the intima of early atherosclerotic lesions of human coronary arteries. Arterioscler Thromb Vasc Biol 1998;18(9):1386–92.

75. Arici M, Walls J. End-stage renal disease, atherosclerosis, and cardiovascular mortality: is C-reactive protein the missing link? Kidney Int 2001;59(2):407–14.

76. Cermak J, Key NS, Bach RR, et al. C-reactive protein induces human peripheral blood monocytes to synthesize tissue factor. Blood 1993;82(2):513–20. Available at: http://www.bloodjournal.org/content/82/2/513. Accessed January 22, 2019.

77. Minami Y, Kajimoto K, Sato N, et al. Effect of elevated C-reactive protein level at discharge on long-term outcome in patients hospitalized for acute heart failure. Am J Cardiol 2018;121(8):961–8.

78. Kim B-S, Jeon DS, Shin MJ, et al. Persistent elevation of C-reactive protein may predict cardiac hypertrophy and dysfunction in patients maintained on hemodialysis. Am J Nephrol 2005;25(3):189–95.

79. Yeun JY, Levine RA, Mantadilok V, et al. C-reactive protein predicts all-cause and cardiovascular mortality in hemodialysis patients. Am J Kidney Dis 2000;35(3):469–76.

80. Chinnappa S, Tu Y-K, Yeh YC, et al. Association between protein-bound uremic toxins and asymptomatic cardiac dysfunction in patients with chronic kidney disease. Toxins (Basel) 2018;10(12). https://doi.org/10.3390/toxins10120520.

81. Lekawanvijit S. Cardiotoxicity of uremic toxins: a driver of cardiorenal syndrome. Toxins (Basel) 2018;10(9). https://doi.org/10.3390/toxins10090352.

82. Lin C-J, Liu H-L, Pan C-F, et al. Indoxyl sulfate predicts cardiovascular disease and renal function deterioration in advanced chronic kidney disease. Arch Med Res 2012;43(6):451–6.

83. Enomoto A, Takeda M, Tojo A, et al. Role of organic anion transporters in the tubular transport of indoxyl sulfate and the induction of its nephrotoxicity. J Am Soc Nephrol 2002;13(7):1711–20.

84. Dou L, Bertrand E, Cerini C, et al. The uremic solutes p-cresol and indoxyl sulfate inhibit endothelial proliferation and wound repair. Kidney Int 2004;65(2):442–51.

85. Wu I-W, Hsu K-H, Lee C-C, et al. p-Cresyl sulphate and indoxyl sulphate predict progression of chronic kidney disease. Nephrol Dial Transplant 2011;26(3):938–47.

86. Han H, Zhu J, Zhu Z, et al. p-Cresyl sulfate aggravates cardiac dysfunction associated with chronic kidney disease by enhancing apoptosis of cardiomyocytes. J Am Heart Assoc 2015;4(6). https://doi.org/10.1161/JAHA.115.001852.

87. Owada S, Goto S, Bannai K, et al. Indoxyl sulfate reduces superoxide scavenging activity in the kidneys of normal and uremic rats. Am J Nephrol 2008;28(3):446–54.

88. Fujii H, Nishijima F, Goto S, et al. Oral charcoal adsorbent (AST-120) prevents progression of cardiac damage in chronic kidney disease through suppression of oxidative stress. Nephrol Dial Transplant 2009;24(7):2089–95.

89. Lekawanvijit S, Krum H. Cardiorenal syndrome: acute kidney injury secondary to cardiovascular disease and role of protein-bound uraemic toxins. J Physiol 2014;592(Pt 18):3969–83.

90. Barreto FC, Barreto DV, Liabeuf S, et al. Serum indoxyl sulfate is associated with vascular disease and mortality in chronic kidney disease patients. Clin J Am Soc Nephrol 2009;4(10):1551–8.

91. Faul C, Amaral AP, Oskouei B, et al. FGF23 induces left ventricular hypertrophy. J Clin Invest 2011;121(11):4393–408.

92. Touchberry CD, Green TM, Tchikrizov V, et al. FGF23 is a novel regulator of intracellular calcium and cardiac contractility in addition to cardiac

hypertrophy. Am J Physiol Endocrinol Metab 2013; 304(8):E863–73.

93. Kao Y-H, Chen Y-C, Lin Y-K, et al. FGF-23 dysregulates calcium homeostasis and electrophysiological properties in HL-1 atrial cells. Eur J Clin Invest 2014;44(8):795–801.

94. Ezekowitz JA, McAlister FA, Armstrong PW. Anemia is common in heart failure and is associated with poor outcomes: insights from a cohort of 12 065 patients with new-onset heart failure. Circulation 2003;107(2):223–5.

95. Palazzuoli A, Antonelli G, Nuti R. Anemia in Cardio-Renal Syndrome: clinical impact and pathophysiologic mechanisms. Heart Fail Rev 2011;16(6): 603–7.

96. Adams KF, Patterson JH, Oren RM, et al. Prospective assessment of the occurrence of anemia in patients with heart failure: results from the study of anemia in a heart failure population (STAMINA-HFP) registry. Am Heart J 2009;157(5):926–32.

97. Young JB, Abraham WT, Albert NM, et al. Relation of low hemoglobin and anemia to morbidity and mortality in patients hospitalized with heart failure (insight from the OPTIMIZE-HF registry). Am J Cardiol 2008;101(2):223–30.

98. McClellan W, Aronoff SL, Bolton WK, et al. The prevalence of anemia in patients with chronic kidney disease. Curr Med Res Opin 2004;20(9): 1501–10.

99. American Journal of Kidney Diseases. KDOQI clinical practice guidelines and clinical practice recommendations for anemia in chronic kidney disease. Am J Kidney Dis 2006;47:S11–5.

100. Grune T, Sommerburg O, Siems WG. Oxidative stress in anemia. Clin Nephrol 2000;53(1 Suppl):S18–22. Available at: http://europepmc.org/abstract/med/10746801. Accessed January 21, 2019.

101. Brezis M, Rosen S. Hypoxia of the renal medulla — its implications for disease. N Engl J Med 1995; 332(10):647–55.

102. Denton KM, Shweta A, Anderson WP. Preglomerular and postglomerular resistance responses to different levels of sympathetic activation by hypoxia. J Am Soc Nephrol 2002; 13(1):27–34. Available at: https://jasn.asnjournals.org/content/13/1/27. Accessed January 21, 2019.

103. Singh AK, Szczech L, Tang KL, et al. Correction of anemia with epoetin alfa in chronic kidney disease. N Engl J Med 2006;355(20):2085–98.

104. Drüeke TB, Locatelli F, Clyne N, et al. Normalization of hemoglobin level in patients with chronic kidney disease and anemia. N Engl J Med 2006;355(20): 2071–84.

105. Pfeffer MA, Burdmann EA, Chen C-Y, et al. A trial of darbepoetin alfa in type 2 diabetes and chronic kidney disease. N Engl J Med 2009;361(21): 2019–32.

106. Swedberg K, Young JB, Anand IS, et al. Treatment of anemia with darbepoetin alfa in systolic heart failure. N Engl J Med 2013;368(13):1210–9.

107. Bouglé A, Duranteau J. Pathophysiology of sepsis-induced acute kidney injury: the role of global renal blood flow and renal vascular resistance. Contrib Nephrol 2011;174:89–97.

108. Mehta RL, Rabb H, Shaw AD, et al. Cardiorenal syndrome type 5: clinical presentation, pathophysiology and management strategies from the eleventh consensus conference of the Acute Dialysis Quality Initiative (ADQI). Contrib Nephrol 2013; 182:174–94.

109. Di Lullo L, Bellasi A, Barbera V, et al. Pathophysiology of the cardio-renal syndromes types 1–5: an uptodate. Indian Heart J 2017;69(2):255–65.

110. Hatamizadeh P, Fonarow GC, Budoff MJ, et al. Cardiorenal syndrome: pathophysiology and potential targets for clinical management. Nat Rev Nephrol 2013;9(2):99–111.

Treatment of Cardiorenal Syndrome

Jack Rubinstein, MD*, Darek Sanford, MD

KEYWORDS

- Cardiorenal syndrome • Systolic dysfunction • Diastolic dysfunction • Heart failure
- Acute kidney injury • Chronic kidney disease • Worsening renal function

KEY POINTS

- There is limited evidence to guide therapies for cardiorenal syndrome; therapies are targeted at symptomatic improvement of heart failure as well as hospital readmissions, morbidity, and mortality in a setting of maintained renal function.
- Diuretics remain the drug of choice for treatment of cardiorenal syndrome with underlying primary cardiac pathologic condition.
- Depending on acuity of insult and extent of renal injury, alternative modalities for treatment include ultrafiltration, peritoneal dialysis, vasodilators, inotrope assistance, and neurohormonal axis inhibition.
- New therapies under investigation, such as vasopressin receptor antagonists, adenosine receptor antagonists, and calcium sensitization, require larger studies to demonstrate benefit in this patient population.

INTRODUCTION

Cardiorenal syndrome (CRS) has long been recognized and generally is identified as a worsening of both cardiac and renal function, which can occur in both the acute and the chronic setting.[1] To simplify and characterize the complex and bidirectional interaction of the heart and kidney, a definition encompassing 5 subtypes reflecting the time frame and principal pathologic condition is most commonly used.[1] Type 1 CRS is exemplified by cardiogenic shock or acute decompensated heart failure (HF), whereby a combination of reduced forward flow and venous congestion lead to acute kidney injury. Worsening renal function (WRF) in this setting is a relatively common occurrence; 1 meta-analysis estimated 25% of patients hospitalized with HF develop WRF, defined as an increase in serum creatinine greater than 0.2 mg/dL. Besides increasing the complexity of managing these patients, incidence as well as the degree of WRF is associated with worsening prognosis, including increased mortality.[2] Risk factors for the development of WRF in HF include elderly age, severe vascular disease, diabetes, hypertension, and prior history of HF and renal dysfunction.[3] As described in later discussion, this category provides a relatively large amount of randomized controlled data from the acute myocardial infarction population as well as patients admitted with a primary diagnosis of HF. Type 2 CRS reflects chronic cardiac dysfunction typified by compensated or acute on chronic HF whereby neurohormonal dysregulation and repeated fluctuation in venous congestion lead to chronic kidney injury. This group is also well represented in the literature, although most end points target mortality, morbidity, and hospital readmissions. Type 3 CRS mirrors type 1 CRS in its timeframe; however, the principal pathologic condition is an acute

Disclosure Statement: The authors have nothing to disclose.
University of Cincinnati, Medical Science Building, 231 Albert Sabin Way, MLC 0542, Cincinnati, OH 45267, USA
* Corresponding author.
E-mail address: rubinsjk@ucmail.uc.edu

Cardiol Clin 37 (2019) 267–273
https://doi.org/10.1016/j.ccl.2019.04.002
0733-8651/19/

worsening in renal function. This type has been found to have a variable impact on cardiac function leading to several sequelae, including arrhythmias, myocardial infarction, and HF. Type 4 CRS comprises the negative impact of chronic kidney disease on cardiac function best illustrated by renal dysfunction leading to uncontrolled hypertension followed by left ventricular hypertrophy and potentially HF with preserved ejection fraction (EF). Type 5 CRS is described best as systemic illness, such as sepsis or lupus, which indirectly or directly leads to both cardiac and renal dysfunction. Most evidenced-based therapies target type 1 and type 2 CRS and are the focus of this article.

DECONGESTION

The acute management of the patient with venous congestion often focuses on the rapid removal of volume to aid in symptomatic relief. There are effective therapies that result in decongestion, although none have been found to improve survival or attenuate disease progression.[4] Likewise, reducing patient sodium intake has been a mainstay of treatment to avoid volume expansion; however, this has never been proven in large randomized trials, and some have even proposed that sodium restriction may have a detrimental effect on outcomes in patients with HF.[5] When considering the clinical presentation of acute decompensated HF with WRF, several pathophysiologic mechanisms have been proposed to the primary nature of kidney injury. Initially, the consensus favored reduced cardiac output or lack of forward flow as the primary driver of kidney injury. Therapies targeting increased contractility as well as vasodilators to reduce both preload and afterload were and are still used in conjunction with diuretics to improve symptoms; however, diuretics alone have not been shown to improve hard cardiac endpoints.[6] Furthermore, the ESCAPE trial aimed to use pulmonary arterial catheters (PAC) in patients with recurrent HF targeting mortality, repeat hospitalization, and symptoms of elevated filling pressures. Although intervention with PAC did not alter these outcomes, unexpectedly, a post hoc analysis of patients revealed baseline right atrial pressure rather than arterial blood flow correlated with baseline serum creatinine, and improving cardiac index did not result in changes to the renal function.[7,8] Thus, the paradigm has shifted toward the concept that venous congestion rather than lack of forward flow as the principal cause of WRF in this population, and at the moment diuretics continue to be the drug of choice for initial treatment of stable patients with type 1 CRS.

Several studies have attempted to establish which, if any, diuretic regimen can be recommended for patients with decompensated HF. The DOSE AHF trial sought to evaluate the effect of diuretic strategy on patient symptoms and renal function over a 72-hour period. Patients received either continuous infusion or bolus diuretic in a low dose (equivalent to prior oral dose) or high dose (2.5 times prior oral dose). No difference was determined between groups; however, the high-dose strategy was associated with greater relief of dyspnea, greater fluid loss and weight loss, and fewer serious adverse events. Although WRF occurred more frequently with the high-dose strategy in the short term, there was no evidence at 60 days of worse clinical outcomes in the high-dose group.[4] Therefore, there are limited data to guide decision making on extent and duration of diuresis in patients hospitalized with HF. A potential marker that has shown promise is hemoconcentration or an increase in both hematocrit and hemoglobin above admission values. When achieved, hemoconcentration has been shown to be associated with increased fluid removal, high-diuretic doses, and reduced body weight, while carrying an increased risk of in-hospital WRF. Even with changes in renal function, hemoconcentration has improved short-term mortality and rates of readmission, suggesting that not all fluctuations in creatinine correlate to a poor prognosis.[9]

Regardless of the diuretic regimen, diuretic resistance is common, especially in patients with severe HF symptoms, and has been reported to occur in 30% of patients with HF on diuretic therapy.[10] No formal definition is available, although the agreed concept is inability to remove volume in a state of venous congestion. Most would agree that inadequate urine output on a regimen of high-dose loop and thiazide diuretics and potentially potassium-sparing diuretics and inotropic agents would constitute diuretic resistance. In this scenario, it is often prudent to consider an alternative modality beyond pharmacologic management for volume removal. One such therapy, ultrafiltration, has been compared with diuretic therapy in patients with decompensated HF in 2 landmark trials. First, UNLOAD showed a reduction in 90-day resource utilization as well as greater weight and fluid loss with no difference in renal function between groups.[11] This study was followed by CARRESS-HF, which unfortunately reported conflicting data. Aggressive pharmacologic therapy, including high doses of intravenous diuretics, titrated to maintain urine output of 3 to 5 L per day combined with intravenous vasodilators and inotropic agents was superior to ultrafiltration, which had a higher incidence of renal injury, adverse events, and no difference in volume removal.[12] In the latest guidelines, ultrafiltration remains a class IIB recommendation for patients with congestion not responding to medical therapy.[13] Last, peritoneal dialysis (PD) has been explored as an alternative to pharmacologic volume removal, although with limited data. Nakayama and colleagues[14] showed in a small study of 12 elderly patients with chronic kidney disease and refractory HF that PD is not only well tolerated but eliminated hospitalization for HF at 2 years.

ENDOGENOUS VASODILATION

As described above, the initial methods for improving outcomes in decompensated HF with type 1 CRS included inotropic agents and vasodilators in an attempt to improve cardiac output, which in theory would increase renal perfusion and facilitate diuresis. Multiple agents have been studied; the most commonly used in this clinical scenario are nitroglycerin and B-type natriuretic peptide (Nesiritide). As an initial strategy in combination with diuretics, these medications were shown to be superior to inotropic agents (primarily dobutamine and dopamine) with lower in-hospital mortality.[6] When compared head to head, Nesiritide demonstrated a more rapid improvement in hemodynamic function and symptom relief, however no difference with respect to serious adverse events or renal function at 30 days.[15] Somewhat contradictory data from the ASCEND HF trial evaluated Nesiritide versus placebo, which found no change in cardiac endpoints, a small but nonsignificant effect on dyspnea, and increased rates of hypotension. Although treatment was not associated with worsening of renal function, increased rates of hypotension were noted; thus, Nesiritide is not recommended for routine use in all-comers with decompensated HF.[16] With regards to renal function, the BNP CARDS trial showed no impact of 48-hour Nesiritide infusion on preservation or improvement in renal function in acute HF.[17] Another failed attempt, the Veritas Trial, aimed to use Tezosentan, an intravenous short-acting endothelial receptor antagonist, with no change in dyspnea and worsening HF death at 7 days.[18] Observational data exist favoring Nitroprusside; however, this is in a specific patient population with low cardiac output and normal or hypertensive blood pressure.[19]

INOTROPIC SUPPORT

When considering the management of cardiogenic shock, inotropic support is critical to maintain perfusion pressure to vital organs, although as clearly shown in the cardiovascular literature, the use of inotropes in this scenario has not been shown to improve outcomes and has frequently been associated with increased mortality.[20–22]

One would surmise this benefit would extend to type 1 CRS; however, it is not until forward flow is severely compromised, cardiac index less than 1.5 L/min/m^2, that renal blood flow begins to decline.[23] This is further corroborated by the findings of the OPTIME CHF trial. Retrospective analysis comparing changes in blood urea nitrogen and estimated glomerular filtration rate to mortality at 60 days in patients with HF treated with Milrinone showed minor improvement in renal function yet no improvement in mortality.[24] Similar findings occurred with evaluation of low-dose dopamine as well as Dobutamine.[20,25] One of the most promising inotropic agents, Levosimendan, both a positive inotropic drug and a vasodilator, has had mixed outcomes in 3 large trials. First, the LIDO trial compared Levosimendan to Dobutamine in patients with severe low-output HF, and a hemodynamic improvement was associated with a lower mortality at 1 and 6 months with Levosimendan.[21] Closely following, the SURVIVE trial again compared Levosimendan to Dobutamine in acute decompensated HF with left ventricular EF less than 30% and found no difference in all-cause mortality at 6 months.[22] Last, REVIVE I and II compared Levosimendan to usual care and found improved symptomatic relief at 5 days; however, this came with increased risk of hypotension, cardiac arrhythmias, and numerically higher risk of death at 90 days.[26]

Although cardiac resynchronization therapy (CRT) is not considered inotropic therapy, it has been proven to increase EF and reduce symptoms in patients with HF. A retrospective analysis of the MIRACLE Study compared patients with normal and reduced renal function. CRT improved New York Heart Association class, EF, and reduced mitral regurgitation as well as increased eGFR in the CKD subset.[27] Although medical inotropic therapy has not been shown to improve renal function in HF, these data suggest that increasing cardiac output can be renoprotective if the unwanted side effects of inotropes can be avoided with a device-based approach.

NEUROHORMONAL AXIS INHIBITION

Preserving both cardiac and renal function during an acute episode of decompensation has also been shown to be critically important in maintaining function long term. Deteriorating renal function has been established to be a poor prognostic sign in patients with HF for decades. Among many studies, a secondary analysis of the DIG trial revealed a clear link between renal dysfunction and mortality in outpatients.[28]

Inhibition of the renal angiotensin aldosterone system (RAAS) is the cornerstone of treatment of HF. One of the first trials to show reduction in mortality with HF, CONSENSUS, added Enalapril, an angiotensin-converting-enzyme inhibitor (ACE-I), to conventional therapy; these deaths were later recognized to be due to lack of progression of HF.[29] Investigation continued with SOLVD again using Enalapril in addition to conventional therapy. Although the baseline serum creatinine cutoff was 2.5 mg/dL, a retrospective analysis showed that use of ACE-I was associated with a reduction of mortality, even in those with severe renal insufficiency.[30] As with diuretics, no dosing guidelines exist, and a typical starting dose is 25% of goal dose with 25% to 50% increases at 4- to 8-week intervals as blood pressure and renal function allow. Safety of this drug class with regards to WRF and hyperkalemia has been well evaluated. An increase of SCr less than 30% of the pretreatment baseline within 2 weeks falls within the normal range.[31] A meta-analysis of 5 placebo-controlled randomized controlled trials (RCT) yielded that, although rates of kidney injury were higher with ACE-I, discontinuation of the drug was infrequent, and even without dose adjustments, renal function returned to baseline.[31] If an increase in SCr greater than 30% is noted, ACE-I should be held, and workup for conditions causing renal hypoperfusion should be initiated. Volume status, vasoconstriction, and renal artery stenosis should be excluded before restarting the medication typically at a lower dose. That being said, ACE-I should be introduced with caution, especially in the setting of WRF because their effect on vasoconstriction of the efferent arteriole can lead to additional decline in function. If serum potassium increases greater than 5.5 mEq, ACE-I dose should be reduced, and the patient medication regimen reviewed for other hyperkalemia-inducing drugs, such as nonsteroidal anti-inflammatory drugs or K-sparing diuretics.[32] RAAS inhibition with ACE-I and/or angiotensin receptor blockers (ARBs) may provide inadequate suppression of aldosterone production during long-term therapy, because both aldosterone and angiotensin II ultimately escape the effects of these drugs, resulting in rebound of aldosterone levels. Aldosterone stimulates sodium and fluid retention and promotes myocardial remodeling and fibrosis as well as endothelial dysfunction and atherosclerosis. Mineralocorticoid receptor antagonism (MRA), in addition to ACE, can provide more complete inhibition of the RAAS, with long-term benefits. However, this comes at a cost of high incidence of hyperkalemia and WRF. Notably, both major trials, Ephesus and RALES, evaluating MRA in HF showed reduction in mortality but excluded patients with SCr greater than 2.5 mg/dL. There are no large-scale RCTs that evaluate the efficacy and safety of MRAs in addition to ACE-Is or ARBs as a treatment strategy for HF in CKD patients. In stage 3 CKD patients with HF, MRA may be considered, but should be used with great caution, limiting the dose to 25 mg/d, and closely monitoring the potassium levels.[33]

Not all facets of the RAAS have shown utility with regards to HF management. Aliskiren, a direct renin inhibitor, had increased rates of hyperkalemia, hypotension, and renal impairment without a reduction in rehospitalization or mortality when added to standard therapy.[34] The new agent, Entresto, a combination of Sacubitril, a neprilysin inhibitor, and Valsartan, an ARB, has been recently added to the list of optimal medical therapy for HF with reduced EF. The Paradigm HF trial compared Entresto to Enalapril and was stopped early due to 20% relative risk reduction in cardiovascular death or hospitalization for HF. No difference in renal function or progression to end-stage renal disease (ESRD) was noted, and post hoc analysis suggested a renoprotective effect for Entresto because the rate of decline of renal function in that group was slower.[35]

Beta-blockade, although counterintuitive, with the goal of increasing forward flow has been shown to improve cardiac outcomes in HF and be renoprotective. In the MERIT trial, Metoprolol succinate with target dose 200 mg daily was added to optimal therapy showing reduction in both worsening HF sudden cardiac deaths.[36] In a secondary analysis dividing patients by renal function, beta-blockade was not only well tolerated across all groups but also found to decrease mortality and hospitalization by 60% in the reduced renal function cohort. Similar findings were noted with the CIBIS II and SENIORS trials, adding Bisoprolol and Nebivolol, respectively, to optimal medical therapy.[37,38] This therapy should be introduced with caution because the side effects of hypotension and bradycardia are poorly tolerated in patients with decompensated HF and may precipitate worsening of symptoms. For patients with ESRD, Carvedilol has been shown to decrease death and hospitalization related to cardiovascular cause.[39]

OTHER THERAPIES

Beyond the traditional medications indicated for HF therapy, several other novel drugs and pathophysiologic mechanisms for kidney injury have been explored. Tolvaptan, a vasopressin V2-receptor antagonist typically used to treat hyponatremia, has been studied for its potential to facilitate diuresis. First, in the ACTIV in CHF trial, Tolvaptan was added to standard therapy to patients admitted with HF. No difference was found in worsening HF, hypokalemia, or renal function at 60 days. A post hoc analysis showed lower mortality in the subgroups of renal dysfunction and severe symptoms.[40] This study was followed by the Everest Trial, which added Tolvaptan to standard therapy for 2 months after being admitted with HF. Over 9 months, no difference in therapy versus placebo was identified, and the conclusion was that Tolvaptan had no effect on hospitalized patients with HF and no effect on long-term mortality.[41] Several trials have evaluated the role of anemia, a known byproduct of chronic renal dysfunction, and the potential for improving outcomes by targeting increased hemoglobin.[42] Unfortunately, Darbepoetin alpha not only has been shown on several occasions to be comparable to placebo but also carries an increased risk of stroke.[43,44] Along this same line, Rolofylline, an A1-Receptor antagonist, has been evaluated without any clinical benefit in HF established to date.[45] Very limited evidence proposes corticosteroids as an adjunct to standard therapy to facilitate diuresis because glucocorticoids can increase natriuretic peptide receptors, leading to effective diuresis and potentially an improvement in renal function.[46] Serelaxin, a recombinant form of human relaxin-2, has properties that allow a reduction in pulmonary capillary wedge pressure and pulmonary artery systolic pressure. Compared with placebo in patients with both reduced EF and preserved EF HF, Serelaxin showed lower incidence of WRF at 48 hours.[47] A high proportion of these patients had hypertension, which may limit the utility of this medication, and more high-quality evaluation is required before further recommendations by guidelines committees.

Novel approaches to the management of diabetes have led to 2 new targets, GLP-1 and SGLT2, which have shown promise both in reduction of HF incidence and in renoprotection.[48,49] Last, a review of urate-lowering therapies showed both an improvement in cardiovascular mortality and mild improvement in renal function for patients with gout treated with Allopurinol or Probenecid.[50,51] Probenecid in particular has been recently shown to have inotropic properties[52] and may be beneficial in a select HF population either as monotherapy or in combination with hydrochlorothiazide in order to enhance diuresis.[53]

REFERENCES

1. Ronco C, Haapio M, House AA, et al. Cardiorenal syndrome. J Am Coll Cardiol 2008;52(19): 1527–39.
2. Damman K, Navis G, Voors AA, et al. Worsening renal function and prognosis in heart failure: systematic review and meta-analysis. J Card Fail 2007; 13(8):599–608.
3. Forman DE, Butler J, Wang Y, et al. Incidence, predictors at admission, and impact of worsening renal function among patients hospitalized with heart failure. J Am Coll Cardiol 2004;43(1):61–7.
4. Felker GM, Lee KL, Bull DA, et al. Diuretic strategies in patients with acute decompensated heart failure. N Engl J Med 2011;364(9):797–805.
5. Doukky MD, Avery E, Mangla A. Impact of dietary sodium restriction on heart failure outcomes. JACC Heart Fail 2016;4(1):24–35.
6. Abraham WT, Adams KF, Fonarow GC, et al. In-hospital mortality in patients with acute decompensated heart failure requiring intravenous vasoactive medications: an analysis from the Acute Decompensated Heart Failure National Registry (ADHERE). J Am Coll Cardiol 2005;45(1):57–64.
7. Binanay C, Califf RM, Hasselblad V, et al. Evaluation study of congestive heart failure and pulmonary artery catheterization effectiveness. JAMA 2005; 294(13):1625–33.
8. Nohria A, Hasselblad V, Stebbins A, et al. Cardiorenal interactions: insights from the ESCAPE trial. J Am Coll Cardiol 2008;51(13):1275–6.
9. Vaduganathan M, Greene SJ, Fonarow GC. Hemoconcentration-guided diuresis in heart failure. Am J Med 2014;12:1154–9.
10. Ravnan SL, Ravnan MC, Deedwania PC. Pharmacotherapy in congestive heart failure: diuretic resistance and strategies to overcome resistance in patients with congestive heart failure. Congest Heart Fail 2002;8:80–5.
11. Costanzo MR, Guglin ME, Saltzberg MT, et al. Ultrafiltration versus intravenous diuretics for patients hospitalized for acute decompensated heart failure. J Am Coll Cardiol 2007;49(6):675–83.
12. Bart BA, Goldsmith SR, Lee KL, et al. Ultrafiltration in decompensated heart failure with cardiorenal syndrome. N Engl J Med 2012;367:2296–304.
13. Yancy CW, Jessup MJ, Bozkurt B, et al. 2013 ACCF/AHA guideline for the management of heart failure. Circulation 2013;128:e240–327.
14. Nakayama M, Nakano M, Nakayama M. Novel therapeutic option for refractory heart failure in elderly patients with chronic kidney disease by incremental peritoneal dialysis. J Cardiol 2010;55:49–54.
15. Publication Committee for the VMAC Investigators (Vasodilatation in the Management of Acute CHF). Intravenous Nesiritide vs nitroglycerin for treatment

of decompensated heart failure: a randomized controlled trial. JAMA 2002;287:1531–40.

16. O'Connor CM, Starling RC, Hernandez AF, et al. Effect of Nesiritide in patients with acute decompensated heart failure. N Engl J Med 2011;365:32–43.

17. Witteles RM, Kao D, Christophers D, et al. Impact of Nesiritide on renal function in patients with acute decompensated heart failure and pre-existing renal dysfunction. J Am Coll Cardiol 2007;50(19): 1835–40.

18. McMurray JJ, Teerlink RJ, Cotter G, et al. Effects of Tezosentan on symptoms and clinical outcomes in patients with acute heart failure. JAMA 2007; 298(17):2009–19.

19. Mullens W, Abrahams Z, Francis GS, et al. Sodium nitroprusside for advanced low-output heart failure. J Am Coll Cardiol 2008;52:200–7.

20. Yamani MH, Haji SA, Starling RC. Comparison of dobutamine-based and milrinone-based therapy for advanced decompensated congestive heart failure: hemodynamic efficacy, clinical outcome, and economic impact. Am Heart J 2001;142(6):998–1002.

21. Follath F, Cleland JG, Just H, et al. Efficacy and safety of intravenous levosimendan compared with dobutamine in severe low-output heart failure (the LIDO study): a randomized double-blind trial. Lancet 2002;360(9328):196–202.

22. Mebazaa A, Nieminen MS, Packer M. Levosimendan vs dobutamine for patients with acute decompensated heart failure. JAMA 2007;297:1883–91.

23. Ljungman S, Laragh JH, Cody RJ. Role of the kidney in congestive heart failure. Relationship of cardiac index to kidney function. Drugs 1990;39(Suppl 4): 10–21.

24. Klein L, Massie B, Leimberger JD, et al. Admission or changes in renal function during hospitalization for worsening heart failure predict postdischarge survival: results from the outcomes of a prospective trial of intravenous milrinone for exacerbations of chronic heart failure (OPTIME-CHF). Circ Heart Fail 2008;1:25–33.

25. Chen HH, Anstrom KJ, Givertz MM, et al. Low-dose dopamine or low-dose Nesiritide in acute heart failure with renal dysfunction. JAMA 2013;310(23): 2533–43.

26. Packer M, Colucci W, Fisher L, et al. Effect of levosimendan on the short-term clinical course of patients with acutely decompensated heart failure. JACC Heart Fail 2013;1:103–11.

27. Boerrigter G, Costello-Boerrigter LC, Abraham WT. Cardiac resynchronization therapy improves renal function in human heart failure with reduced glomerular filtration rate. J Card Fail 2008;14(7):539–46.

28. Shlipak MG, Smith GL, Rathore SS. Renal function, digoxin therapy, and heart failure outcomes: evidence from the digoxin intervention group trial. J Am Soc Nephrol 2004;15:2195–203.

29. CONSENSUS Trial Study Group. Effects of Enalapril on mortality in severe congestive heart failure. N Engl J Med 1987;316:1429–35.

30. Yusuf S, Pitt B, Davis CE, et al. Effect of Enalapril on survival in patients with reduced left ventricular ejection fractions and congestive heart failure. N Engl J Med 1991;325(5):293–302.

31. Valika AA, Gheorghiade M. ACE inhibitor therapy for heart failure in patients with impaired renal function: a review of the literature. Heart Fail Rev 2013;18(2): 135–40.

32. Liu PP. Cardiorenal syndrome in heart failure: a cardiologist's perspective. Can J Cardiol 2008; 24(Suppl B):25B–9B.

33. Albaghdadi M, Gheorghiade M. Mineralocorticoid receptor antagonism: therapeutic potential in acute heart failure syndromes. Eur Heart J 2011;32(21): 2626–33.

34. McMurray JJ, Packer M, Desai AS. Angiotensin-neprilysin inhibition versus Enalapril in heart failure. N Engl J Med 2014;371:993–1004.

35. Gheorghiade M, Bohm M, Greene SJ, et al. Effect of Aliskiren on post-discharge mortality and heart failure readmissions among patients hospitalized for heart failure. JAMA 2013;309(11):1125–35.

36. Goldstein S, Fagerberg B, Hjalmarson A. Metoprolol controlled release/extended release in patients with severe heart failure: analysis of the experience in the MERIT-HF study. J Am Coll Cardiol 2001;38(4): 932–8.

37. The cardiac insufficiency bisprolol study II (CIBIS II): a randomized trial. Lancet 1999;353(9146):9–13.

38. Flather MD, Shibata MC, Coats AJ. Randomized trial to determine the effect of nebivolol on mortality and cardiovascular admission in elderly patients with heart failure (SENIORS). Eur Heart J 2005;26(3): 215–25.

39. Cice G, Ferrara L, D'Andrea A, et al. Carvedilol increases two-year survivalin in dialysis patients with dilated cardiomyopathy: a prospective, placebo-controlled trial. J Am Coll Cardiol 2003;41(9): 1438–44.

40. Gheorghiade M, Gattis WA, O'Connor CM, et al. Effects of Tolvaptan, a vasopressin antagonist, in patients hospitalized with worsening heart failure. JAMA 2004;291:1963–71.

41. Konstam MA, Gheorghiade M, Burnett JC, et al. Effects of oral Tolvaptan in patients hospitalized for worsening heart failure. JAMA 2007;297:1319–31.

42. Palazzuoli A, Ruocco G, Pellegrini M. The role of erythropoietin stimulating agents in anemic patients with heart failure: solved and unresolved questions. Ther Clin Risk Management 2014;10:641–50.

43. Ghali JK, Anand IS, Abraham WT, et al. Randomized double-blind trial of darbepoetin alfa in patients with symptomatic heart failure. Circulation 2008;117(4): 526–35.

44. Swedberg K, Young JB, Anand IS. Treatment of anemia with darbeopotein alfa in systolic heart failure. N Engl J Med 2013;368:1210–9.

45. Massie BM, O'Connor CM, Metra M, et al. Rolofylline, an adenosine A1-receptor antagonist, in acute heart failure. N Engl J Med 2010;363:1419.

46. Liu C, Liu K. Effects of glucocorticoids in potentiating diuresis in heart failure patients with diuretic resistance. J Card Fail 2014;20(9):625–9.

47. Metra M, Cotter G, Davison BA, et al. Effect of Serelaxin on cardiac, renal, and hepatic biomarkers in the relaxin in acute heart failure (RELAX-AHF) development program: correlation with outcomes. J Am Coll Cardiol 2013;16(2):196–206.

48. Zinman B, Wanner C, Lachin J, et al. Empagliflozin, cardiovascular outcomes, and mortality in type 2 diabetes. N Engl J Med 2015;373:2117–28.

49. Scheen A. GLP-1 receptor agonists and heart failure in diabetes. Diabetes Metab 2017;43:2813–9.

50. Richette P, Latourte A, Bardin T. Cardiac and renal protective effects of urate-lowering therapy. Rheumatology 2018;57:i47–50.

51. Kim S, Neogi T, Kang E, et al. Cardiovascular risks of probenecid versus allopurinol in older patients with Gout. J Am Coll Cardiol 2018;71(9):994–1004.

52. Robbins N, Gilbert M, Kumar M, et al. Probenecid improves cardiac function in patients with heart failure with reduced ejection fraction in vivo and cardiomyocyte calcium sensitivity in vitro. J Am Heart Assoc 2018;7:e007148.

53. Barone S, Xu J, Zahedi K. Probenecid pre-treatment downregulates the kidney Cl/HCO3 exchanger (pendrin) and potentiates hydrochlorothiazide-induced diuresis. Front Physiol 2018;9:849.

Hypertensive Emergencies
A Review of Common Presentations and Treatment Options

Latoya Brathwaite, MD*, Max Reif, MD

KEYWORDS

• Hypertensive crisis • Hypertensive urgency • Hypertensive emergency • End-organ damage

KEY POINTS

• Severe hypertension is a systolic blood pressure greater than 180 mm Hg or a diastolic blood pressure greater than 120 mm Hg.
• It is classified as hypertensive urgency (without end-organ damage) and hypertensive emergency (with end-organ damage).
• An acute increase in blood pressure may also lead to end-organ damage before achieving the blood pressure threshold of greater than 180/120 mm Hg.
• Treatment includes a careful 10% to 15% decrease in blood pressure in the first of hour of treatment and 25% decrease with in the first 2 hours of treatment.
• The antihypertensive needed depends on the type of end-organ damage, the drug's pharmacokinetics, and the patient's comorbidities.

INTRODUCTION

Hypertension is very prevalent. The 2017 American College of Cardiology/American Heart Association Task Force on Clinical Practice guidelines of lowered the blood pressure level that defines hypertension to 120/80 mm Hg or above.[1] This has caused the prevalence in the United States to increase to 46% of the adult population (from 32% according to the older definition of 140/90 mm Hg).[1] It must be kept in mind that blood pressure increases generally with age, and that the prevalence is greater in the older segments of the population.[2,3] As age increases, there is a near parallel increase in systolic blood pressure.[4] As antihypertensive therapy has become more widely used, chronic, untreated hypertension has become a less common cause of hypertensive emergencies. At present, about 85% of adults are aware of their elevated blood pressure, 80% are being treated, and about 70% are controlled.[1]

Despite the improvement in hypertension control, hypertensive emergencies remain a serious clinical challenge. The frequency of hypertensive emergencies varies with the population under study. In one European study, about 47.22% of emergency room visits were due to severe hypertension.[5] The average age of patients admitted to the hospital with hypertensive emergency is between 55 and 60 years old.[5,6] The incidence is higher in African Americans, but the overall frequency is not much different in the United States.[6]

DEFINITIONS

Several definitions have been used to classify severe hypertension and hypertensive emergencies. The terms "hypertensive urgency," "hypertensive crisis," and "malignant hypertension" are confusing and the authors prefer to use the terms "uncontrolled severe hypertension" for cases without acute target organ damage and

University of Cincinnati Medical Center, Medical Sciences Building, Room 6102, 231 Albert Sabin Way, Cincinnati, OH 45267, USA
* Corresponding author.
E-mail address: brathwla@ucmail.uc.edu

Cardiol Clin 37 (2019) 275–286
https://doi.org/10.1016/j.ccl.2019.04.003
0733-8651/19/© 2019 Elsevier Inc. All rights reserved.

"hypertensive emergency" for conditions when acute target organ damage or the risk of severe immediate complications are present. The level of blood pressure of greater than 180/120 mm Hg to define "severe hypertension" is arbitrary, but can be helpful to alert the physician to assess causes, presence of end-organ damage and possible therapies.

Not all patients who present with severe elevation of blood pressure require immediate hospitalization and intravenous therapy. It is important to assess the clinical context of the severe hypertension and to distinguish between situations that show manifestations of acute target organ damage or danger of complications, and situations that can be managed conservatively, usually with oral agents.

Commonly used terms and definitions

- Hypertensive crisis has been used to include all clinical presentations with an elevated blood pressure with a systolic blood pressure of greater than 180 mm Hg and a diastolic blood pressure of greater than 120 mm Hg with or without signs of end-organ damage.
- Hypertensive urgency has been described having an elevated blood pressure with systolic a blood pressure of greater than 180 mm Hg and a diastolic blood pressure of greater than 120 mm Hg without signs of end-organ damage. Patients can present with symptoms of headache, anxiety, pain, and upset stomach, which may lead to worsened hypertension and not be the cause.

- Hypertensive emergency is an elevated blood pressure with a systolic blood pressure of greater than 180 mm Hg and a diastolic blood pressure of greater than 120 mm Hg with signs of end-organ damage.

PATHOPHYSIOLOGY

In 1949, concept of a mosaic theory was introduced to explain the etiology of hypertension. Hypertension was theorized to be related to chemical, neural, vascular elasticity, cardiac output, blood viscosity, vascular caliber, volume, and reactivity effects on tissue perfusion pressure and resistance.[7] Hypertension is not a single disease, but a heterogenous group of disorders with discrete etiologies[8] that leads to the phenotype expressed as sustained elevated blood pressure.[7] Technically, blood pressure can be represented as the mean arterial pressure defined as cardiac output as it relates to total vascular resistance (blood pressure = cardiac output × total vascular resistance). There are many factors that affect these components that can upset this balance.

When the elevation of blood pressure reaches a critical level (often around 180/120 mm Hg), the vascular myogenic response increases vascular resistance. The myogenic response is vascular vasoconstriction in response to an increase in intravascular pressure.[9] The relative peripheral hypoperfusion causes an increase in vasoactive hormones, such as angiotensin II, norepinephrine, endothelin, and antidiuretic hormone.[3] This maladaptive response worsens the peripheral resistance and leads to a vicious cycle (Fig. 1). Elevated pressure causes endothelial damage,

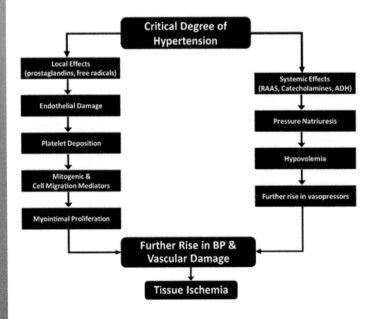

Fig. 1. Pathogenesis of malignant hypertension. ADH, antidiuretic hormone; BP, blood pressure; RAAS, renin–angiotensin–aldosterone system.

platelet and fibrin deposition, and arterial fibrinoid necrosis. The production of nitric oxide is impaired. The vascular damage further impairs perfusion, with resulting myointimal proliferation, fluid extravasation, and tissue infarction. If left unchecked, this process leads to permanent organ damage and death. The organs most often affected are the brain, heart, large arteries, and kidneys.[10–12] With appropriate treatment, the cycle of vasoconstriction–ischemia–vasoconstriction can be broken, with dramatic improvements in outcomes (see **Fig. 1**).

The kidney plays a big role in blood pressure regulation through the renin–angiotensin system and pressure natriuresis. There are several entities that leads to the release of renin from the renal afferent arteriole not limited to decreased perfusion pressure, decreased sodium delivery and beta-adrenergic receptor stimulation. This triggers a cascade of reactions that leads to the conversion of angiotensinogen to angiotensin II. Angiotensin II is a potent pressor that leads to an increase in vascular resistance and production of proinflammatory cytokines through the stimulation of angiotensin II type 1 receptor.[3,10] The end of the pathway leads to the production of aldosterone leading to sodium and water retention.[3]

An increase in blood pressure causes an increase in renal sodium excretion over hours to days (pressure natriuresis). There is also an increase in nitric oxide, prostaglandin E2, and kinins release with a decrease in angiotensin II production.[13] This process is impaired in states of reduced glomerular filtration rate and leads to chronically elevated levels of angiotensin II. The inability to excrete sodium normally can contribute to volume overload and further increases in blood pressure.

RISK FACTORS

Hypertension is the most modifiable risk factor affecting cardiovascular disease and stroke and contributors of premature morbidity and mortality.[3,6] Long-standing primary hypertension, especially when undertreated or untreated, has the potential of becoming more severe and evolving into a hypertensive emergency. Hypertensive emergency risk factors include:

- Female sex,
- Obesity,
- Presence of hypertensive or coronary heart disease,
- A higher number of prescribed antihypertensive drugs, and
- Nonadherence to medication.[14,15]

Renal disease increases the risk of developing severe hypertension and hypertension can worsen renal disease. Intrarenal vascular damage has the potential of reducing the glomerular filtration rate and worsening proteinuria and renal artery disease can lead to renovascular hypertension and ischemic nephropathy.

African American adults have among the highest prevalence of hypertension in the world. In the United States, nearly 1 out of 3 adults have elevated blood pressure, with the highest rates among African Americans followed by non-Hispanic whites.[3,6] Among non-Hispanic black men and women, the age-adjusted prevalence of hypertension was 44.9% and 46.1%, respectively.[16] Although men develop hypertension at an earlier age, women are more likely to have a cardiovascular event when compared with men.[3]

Patients who experience a hypertensive emergency incur an increase in short- and intermediate-term risk for mortality after adjusting for age, sex, and ethnicity.[17] Environmental factors that can contribute include salt intake, obesity, and a sedentary lifestyle.[17] Dyslipidemia, hyperglycemia, and lower renal function was associated with a high prevalence of hypertensive emergency when compared with hypertensive urgency, controlled hypertensive and normotensive patients.[18] **Box 1** lists the risk factors for a hypertensive emergency.

CLINICAL FEATURES

Hypertensive emergencies are characterized by acute or impending organ damage, usually described in the setting of systolic and diastolic blood pressures greater than 180/120 mm Hg.

Box 1
Risk factors for hypertensive emergency

Long-standing hypertension

Preoperative or postoperative hypertension

Renal disease

Stroke

Head trauma

Eclampsia

Cocaine or similar drugs

Acute withdrawal of beta-blockers or centrally acting drugs like clonidine

Treatment with vascular endothelial growth factor

Pheochromocytoma

This can be misleading because end-organ damage can be seen at lower levels.[19] Instead, it the rate of rise that is important.[2,3,19] A previously normotensive patient may experience end-organ damage before reaching that threshold and a chronically hypertensive person can tolerate higher blood pressure levels. As a result, patients presenting with an elevated blood pressure without a previous history of elevated blood pressures should be assessed for signs of end-organ damage.[2] Organ systems that can be affected include central nervous, cardiovascular, pulmonary, renal, and adrenal systems.

The evaluation should include a full history, which includes pain evaluation (location, quality, radiation, duration), presence of shortness of breath, mental status history to assess acute mental status changes, hypertensive encephalopathy, illicit drug use, and previous diagnosis of hypertension, its control, and adherence to medications. The physical examination should include an accurate blood pressure measurement, funduscopic examination looking for papilledema, acute hemorrhages, or exudates; neurologic examination to assess for a cerebrovascular accident; a full cardiac and pulmonary examination to assess for findings consistent with heart failure (lower extremity swelling, positive hepatojugular reflux, new murmurs); aortic dissection (unequal blood pressures); and fluid overload. If the examination is not clear and there is concern for undiagnosed organ damage, radiologic imaging maybe needed for further evaluation. An electrocardiogram can check for signs of cardiac dysfunction. Laboratory tests should include a renal panel to assess for renal dysfunction; a complete blood count to assess for anemia and thrombocytopenia; and a peripheral smear to look for schistocytes and lactic dehydrogenase levels to assess for microangiopathic hemolytic anemia. The lactic acid level can represent decreased perfusion. A urine drug screen rules out the use of common illicit drugs like cocaine and PCP. Finally, a pregnancy test can rule out preeclampsia for undiagnosed pregnancies.

Intracerebral hypertension can cause retinal hemorrhages and papilledema. Papilledema is often associated with hypertensive encephalopathy, but either feature can occur without the other. Acute coronary syndromes can precipitate a hypertensive emergency, but in turn can also be the result of severely elevated blood pressure. Pulmonary edema owing to left ventricular failure can elevate blood pressure and the increased afterload impairs left ventricular performance further.

GOALS OF THERAPY

The first step after the initial assessment of the patient is to determine if there is acute or impending target organ damage. In a case of a true hypertensive emergency, elevated blood pressure with signs of end-organ damage, immediate therapy with intravenous agents is mandatory because they are short acting, easily and readily titratable.[3,20] Whenever available, admission to an intensive care unit and intraarterial pressure monitoring should be started to avoid excessive lowering of blood pressure because that can also lead to end-organ damage, namely, strokes.

In most cases, a lowering of the mean arterial blood pressure by at most 10% to 15% within the first hour and 25% with in the first 2 hours is adequate and should only be exceeded in special situations, such as aortic dissection, eclampsia, or pheochromocytoma crisis.[1] Once the vicious cycle of vasoconstriction and hypoperfusion is broken, the blood pressure can then be lowered more gradually and medications can be switched from the intravenous to the oral route. The choice of the antihypertensive agents should be based on the type of end-organ damage, the drugs pharmacokinetics, and the patient's comorbidities.[1,3]

Of note, the arterial changes of severe hypertension are partially reversible with time. In a hypertensive emergency, a careful but immediate decrease of the blood pressure is paramount and a workup for secondary causes of hypertension should never delay treatment.

To date, there are no large, randomized, controlled trials with a comprehensive evaluation of antihypertensive to reduce morbidity or mortality in patients with hypertensive emergencies. This lack of high-grade evidence is related to the small size of trials, the lack of long-term follow-up, and failure to report outcomes.

SPECIFIC CLINICAL SITUATIONS

Owing to the heterogeneity of hypertensive emergency, there are specific clinical situations that have special pathophysiology and management. These concerns will be addressed in this section. **Table 1** lists medications to consider for hypertensive emergency management and special considerations are discussed here.

Hypertensive Encephalopathy

The brain has a great capacity to autoregulate its blood flow. Cerebral blood flow remains constant over a wide range of systemic blood pressure levels. In individuals with chronically elevated blood pressure, there is autoregulatory

Table 1
IV medications that can be used in hypertensive emergency

Drug 81 Focused	Dosage	Onset (min)	Duration	Comments
Nitrates				
Sodium nitroprusside	0.5 µg/kg/min, increase 0.5 µg/kg/min every 20–60 min	<2	1–10 min	Uses: Acute coronary syndrome, heart failure, aortic dissection, blood pressure control after surgery. Avoid in renal insufficiency owing to the risk of cyanide toxicity.
Nitroglycerin	5 µg/min, increase by 5 µg/kg/min every 3–5 min; max 20 µg/min	Immediate	3–5 min	Uses: Acute coronary syndrome, heart failure, preeclampsia. Avoid in hypovolemia. Use with caution in head injury or use of phosphodiesterase-5 inhibitors like sildenafil (Viagra).
Calcium channel blocker				
Clevidipine	1–2 mg/h then titrate to 4–6 mg/h	2–4	5–15 min	Uses: Acute coronary syndrome, postoperative hypertension especially cardiac surgery, acute renal failure, aortic dissection, sympathetic crisis, cerebrovascular accident. It is a very short acting third-generation dihydropyridine that leads to coronary vasodilation while maintaining splanchnic and renal blood flow. Titration may double every 90 s to goal blood pressure. Every 1–2 mg/h increase relates to a 2–4 mm Hg systolic blood pressure reduction.
Nicardipine	5 mg/h then increase by 2.5 mg/h every 15 min to max of 15 mg/h	10	<8 h	Uses: Acute coronary syndrome, aortic dissection, acute renal failure, sympathetic crisis, cerebrovascular accident. It is a second-generation dihyropyridine that acts as a vasodilator. Reduce at rate of 3 mg/h after goal is achieved

(continued on next page)

Table 1
(continued)

Drug 81 Focused	Dosage	Onset (min)	Duration	Comments
Dopamine 1 agonist				
Fenoldopam	0.1–0.3 µg/kg/min increasing by 0.05–0.1 µg/kg/min every 15 min to goal	10	1 h	Uses: Hypertension in setting of acute kidney injury, cerebrovascular accident. It is a peripheral dopamine receptor agonist the leads to renal artery vasodilation. Start with low initial dose to prevent reflex tachycardia. Use for up to 48 h.
Adrenergic blocking agents				
Labetalol	Bolus 10–20 mg then infuse 2 mg/min to max of 6 mg/min	2–5	2–18 h (dose dependent)	Uses: Aortic dissection, acute coronary syndrome, preeclampsia/eclampsia, cerebrovascular accident. It is a combined alpha-1 adrenergic nonselective beta-adrenergic receptor blocker. It maintains cerebral, renal and coronary blood flow. Do not stop abruptly.
Esmolol	Initial bolus: 1,000 mcg/kg over 30 seconds, followed by a 150 mcg/kg/minute infusion	2–10	10–30 min	Uses: Aortic dissection, acute coronary syndrome. Can be used for intraoperative and postoperative care.
Other agents				
Hydralazine	Preeclampsia/eclampsia: 5 mg/dose then 5–10 mg every 20–30 min as needed; Hypertension: IV 10–20 mg/dose every 4–6 h as needed to max of 40 mg/dose.	5–20	1–4 h depending on whether patient is a fast or slow acetylator	It is a short-acting arterial vasodilator and increases renal blood flow.
Enalaprilat	IV dose 1.25 mg over a 5-min period every 6 h	15–30	6–12 h	Uses: Heart failure, Slow onset, long duration
Phentolamine	5–20 mg for hypertensive crisis titrate by 5 mg every 1–2 h; surgery for pheochromocytoma: 5 mg max dose 1–2 h before procedure, repeat as needed every 2–4 h until goal	Immediate	15–30 min	Uses: Pheochromocytoma related hypertension. Monoamine oxidase inhibitor interactions, cocaine, amphetamine use.

Abbreviations: IV, intravenous; max, maximum; min, minimum.
Data from Refs.[1,3,33]

adaptation. This adaptation explains why chronic hypertensives will tolerate a much higher blood pressure when compared with young and/or previously normotensive individuals.

When the blood pressure exceeds the upper limit of the autoregulatory capacity, the cerebral arteries dilate, first in the less muscular segments and later diffusely. The brain becomes hyperperfused with leakage of intravascular fluid into brain tissue and increased intracerebral pressure. The symptoms of hypertensive encephalopathy are diverse: headache, vomiting, confusion, visual disturbances, and coma. A computed tomography scan or MRI shows edema mostly in the parietooccipital regions, but it can also affect the cerebellum and the frontal areas of the brain. These diffuse findings explain the protean nature of the symptoms.

The diagnosis of hypertensive encephalopathy is one of exclusion. It can be difficult to distinguish a cerebrovascular accident from a purely hypertensive event. Several conditions can mimic or coexist with hypertensive encephalopathy. Conditions like end-stage renal disease and cerebrovascular accidents can cause severely elevated blood pressures and cause altered mental status independently. As a result, controlling the blood pressure will not completely reverse the altered mental status. In contrast, the initiation of hypertensive treatment in hypertensive encephalopathy resolves symptoms quickly.

Nitroprusside is an effective antihypertensive agent with a rapid onset of action and easy titratability. It is a potent arterial and venous vasodilator, but is not optimal in cases of cerebral edema. Current recommendations give preference to nicardipine and labetalol.[21] If central nervous system symptoms do not resolve or worsen with treatment, the level of blood pressure reduction must be lessened until symptoms improve. This measure will exclude hypertensive encephalopathy as the diagnosis.

Posterior reversible encephalopathy syndrome can present as a hypertensive emergency. Posterior reversible encephalopathy syndrome is a clinical radiographic syndrome characterized by symptoms including a headache, seizures, altered consciousness, and visual disturbances.[22] Diagnosis depends on clinical presentation and MRI findings consistent with vasogenic edema localized in the posterior cerebral hemisphere.[6] The pathophysiology is not clearly understood, but 1 theory proposes increased hydrostatic pressure that leads to cerebral vasogenic edema and systemic inflammation. Uremia or supratherapeutic levels of immunosuppressive therapy like cyclosporine and tacrolimus may be contributing factors.[7,8,23] Withdrawal or decreased dosing of these medications has resulted in improved symptoms.[7]

Stroke

The presence of a stroke, whether hemorrhagic or embolic, must be evaluated. A stroke reduces the brains' autoregulatory ability and makes the patient more vulnerable to rapid changes in blood pressure. As a result, blood pressure lowering in cases of stroke differs from the management of hypertensive encephalopathy. Acute cerebrovascular accidents often present with increased blood pressures. Acute ischemic stroke usually does not require blood pressure reduction, unless the patient is being considered for tissue plasminogen activator therapy and the blood pressure is greater than 185/110 mm Hg. If the blood pressure exceeds 220/110 mm Hg, it is recommended to lower the mean arterial pressure by 15% during the first 24 hours.[1] As of the 2018, according to the American Heart Association/American Stroke Association guidelines, there are no studies that address hypotension in patients with an acute stroke.[20]

A hemorrhagic stroke can be accompanied by elevation of blood pressure owing to sympathetic overactivity. The excess catecholamines may decrease over the next few hours, and blood pressure may drop spontaneously. Several randomized trials have examined the effects of more aggressive lowering of blood pressure. In any case of stroke, the cerebral autoregulation can be impaired, and blood pressure lowering carries the risk of increasing the extent of ischemic brain tissue. The current American Stroke Association guideline for acute intracranial hemorrhage recommends a goal blood pressure of 140 mm Hg systolic as safe.[21,24] This recommendation was based INTERACT-2 and ATACH-2 trials, which showed a marginal benefit in decreasing the size of the hematoma and mortality at 90 days with the goal of 140 mm Hg systolic.[25,26] A systolic blood pressure of less than 140 mm Hg was associated with an increase in adverse renal outcomes.[26] The 2018 European Society of Cardiology/European Society of Hypertension Guidelines published since the above studies do not recommend lowering blood pressure in patients with an acute hemorrhagic stroke unless the systolic blood pressure is greater than 220 mm Hg.[27]

Current guidelines for cerebrovascular accidents recommend the use of intravenous agents such as labetalol, nicardipine, and clevidipine to safely lower blood pressure without increasing the intracranial pressure.[21,28]

Cardiovascular Disease

Long-standing primary hypertension leads to arteriolosclerosis and accelerated atherosclerosis.[29] The increased peripheral vascular resistance will eventually cause left ventricular hypertrophy and, if unchecked, congestive heart failure. In cases of severe left ventricular failure, volume overload and low blood pressure often dominate the clinical picture, but in some cases pain and anxiety can elevate blood pressure. If the left ventricle is able to generate enough pressure, the state of a hypertensive emergency can be reached. The stress-induced high catecholamine levels are usually marked by tachycardia.[30,31]

Acute coronary syndromes can have a very similar presentation. In that situation, rapid lowering of the blood pressure and of the heart rate are indicated. In addition to oxygen and morphine, nitroprusside and nitroglycerin are good choices, but require intraarterial monitoring. Intravenous nitrates reduce peripheral vascular resistance and improve coronary perfusion and myocardial oxygen consumption. Sodium nitroprusside may cause a coronary flow steal mechanism caused by generalized coronary vasodilation and should be avoided.[32] Beta-blockers lower the heart rate, but can depress left ventricular function and have to be used with caution. Nitrates given to patients on sildenafil or other phosphodiesterase type 5 inhibitors for pulmonary hypertension can cause profound hypotension. Unlike pure beta-adrenergic blocking agents that decrease cardiac output (eg, esmolol), labetalol maintains cardiac output as well as the cerebral, renal, and coronary blood flow.[33] Diuretics should be reserved for states of hypervolemia and pulmonary edema. A precipitous decrease in blood pressure after the initiation of intravenous antihypertensives can occur in patients who are hypovolemic. The systolic blood pressure should not be lowered to less than 100 mm Hg to avoid coronary hypoperfusion. Left ventricular function often improves rapidly with reduction of both preload and afterload.

For acute aortic syndromes, a delay in recognition, diagnosis, or treatment carries a high mortality. As a result, it is important to identify risk factors. Uncontrolled hypertension is the most modifiable risk factor. Other risk factors are pregnancy, connective tissue disorders, congenital aortopathy history, and bicuspid aortic valves.[33] A classic presentation includes a sudden onset of severe chest pain that radiates to the neck or jaw in ascending dissection or to the back in descending dissection. Chest radiographs, computed tomography scan, MRI, or a transesophageal echocardiogram may be needed to establish diagnosis if there is clinical suspicion.[33,34] A computed tomography scan is preferred owing to ease of accessibility and image quality.[33,35] First-line therapy includes rapid-acting intravenous beta-blockers like labetalol or esmolol for a blood pressure goal of 100 and 120 mm Hg systolic and less than or equal to 60 to 70 mm Hg diastolic.[3] Aortic dissection requires immediate and aggressive reduction in blood pressure and (if appropriate) heart rate. Beta-blockers such as esmolol or labetalol are good choices. If needed, nicardipine or nitroprusside can be added based on their mechanism of action.

Clevidipine was found to be equivalent to nitroglycerin, sodium nitroprusside, and nicardipine for the management of acute hypertension treatment in cardiac surgery patients in the ESCAPE trials I and II.[36] Angiotensin-converting enzyme (ACE) inhibitors like enalaprilat have been shown to be beneficial in heart failure, but are is not recommended owing to the potential for renal failure in patients in this acute setting and population.[20,37] Sodium nitroprusside, a first-choice agent for the majority of hypertensive emergencies, is an arterial and venous vasodilator that decreases both afterload and preload.[33] However, it should be avoided if there is renal insufficiency and neurologic symptoms. Nitroglycerin is great for ischemic heart disease and after a coronary bypass because it reduces preload, increases coronary blood flow, suppresses coronary vasospasm, and decreases cardiac oxygen demands. Nicardipine increase both stroke volume and coronary blood flow with a favorable effect on myocardial oxygen balance.[33] This property is useful in patients with coronary artery disease and systolic heart failure. First-generation calcium channel blockers have a negative inotropic effect. Second-generation calcium channel blockers showed beneficial hemodynamics, but no improvement on survival.[38] Highlights of common parenteral drugs used in the treatment are provided in **Table 1**.

Kidney Disease and Renovascular Hypertension

Hypertension has been reported in 67% to 92% of patients with chronic kidney disease, with an increasing prevalence as kidney function declines. Patients who were admitted with decompensated heart failure that incurred both a sustained and transient acute kidney injury had a significant increased risk of readmission with in 30 days.[39,40] A case series included 12 patients who were diagnosed as having hypertensive emergencies and underwent renal biopsies. Collapse of the glomeruli was found in all 12 patients. In 9 patients, the mean creatinine level decreased significantly from 6.68 ± 5.30 (range, 2.1–18.5 mg/dL) to 2.69 ± 1.20 (range, 1.4–5.4 mg/dL). One patient had a repeat biopsy 12 months after blood pressure control that showed resolution of the onion skin pattern in the patient's arterioles.[41] This report illustrates that the effects of hypertension can be reversible with treatment.

For chronic hypertensive treatment, adults with chronic kidney disease complicated by proteinuria (as defined by albuminuria >300 mg/d or mg/g albumin to creatinine ratio), it is recommended to start with an ACE inhibitor or an angiotensin receptor blocker. If the patient has nephrotic range proteinuria ($\geq$ 3 g/d), the blood pressure goal is less than 120/80 mm Hg as tolerated. If there is no proteinuria, the initiation of first line agents are appropriate. First-line agents include:

- Thiazide diuretics,
- Calcium channel blockers,
- ACE inhibitors, and
- Angiotensin receptor blockers.

The blood pressure goal is less than 130/80 mm Hg.[1] Renin–angiotensin–aldosterone system (RAAS) blockade medications should generally not be used in setting of hypertensive emergency owing to increased risk of developing an acute kidney injury.

As chronic kidney disease worsens (stage $\geq$4) or in the setting of hypoalbuminemia, the effect of diuretics decreases. Thiazide diuretics are changed to or added to loop diuretics. It is also important to focus on nonpharmaceutical options like salt reduction and secondary causes like obesity and obstructive sleep apnea.[42]

Renal artery stenosis can present with hypertensive emergency, flash pulmonary edema, and acute kidney injury or progression of chronic kidney disease. Atherosclerotic disease is the most common cause of renal artery stenosis, and nonatherosclerotic disease accounts for approximately 10% (mostly fibromuscular dysplasia).[1] Fibromuscular dysplasia usually affects women aged between 30 and 50 years of age.

Screening tests include magnetic resonance angiography, helical computed tomographic angiography, doppler ultrasound examination, renal scintigraphy (ie, captopril scan), invasive angiography, peripheral renin levels, and renal vein renin sampling. Doppler ultrasound examination is easily obtained, safe, and inexpensive. As a result, it is usually the first screening test used. However, its accuracy depends on operator experience, which leads to 60% to 90% accuracy. Aside from invasive renal arteriography, magnetic resonance angiography has the highest sensitivity and specificity of 90% to 100%. A decrease in renal function after initiation of an ACE inhibitor or angiotensin receptor blocker is often associated with bilateral RAAS, but does not give a definitive diagnosis. In the setting of blood pressure that can be controlled medically and chronic kidney disease, if advanced, medical therapy is preferred to revascularization. Revascularization can be considered if it is due to fibromuscular dysplasia or in atherosclerotic renal artery stenosis when medical management of hypertension has failed and there is hope that it would stabilize renal function or heart failure.[43]

Hydralazine is a short-acting arterial vasodilator and increased renal blood flow.[44] Fenoldopam is a peripheral dopamine 1 receptor that leads to renal artery vasodilation. It is metabolized by the liver without cytochrome P450 enzyme involvement. It leads to natriuresis and increase urine output.[45] Nicardipine is a second generation dihydropyridine which acts as a vasodilator. Though it does not specifically have renal activity, it has been showed through various trials to be effective in blood pressure reduction.[46] The CLUE study subanalysis showed that patients with eGFR less than 75 ml/min were more likely to reach their blood pressure goals with in 30 mins compared with labetalol.[47] Clevidipine is a very short acting third generation dihydropyridine which is metabolized by RBC esterases.[3] It is a direct coronary vasodilator, increases cardiac output, stroke volume while maintaining splanchnic and renal blood flow.[3] Finally, Nitroprusside is both an arterial and venous dilator which should be avoided in patients with impaired renal function as it can lead to cyanide toxicity.[48]

Scleroderma

Scleroderma renal crisis is a complication of scleroderma that carries high morbidity and mortality. It usually presents with an abrupt increase in blood pressure in relation to the baseline blood pressure and acute kidney injury. The clinical picture is one of hypertensive emergency with arterial changes that resemble other forms of hypertensive vascular disease. Kidney biopsy typically shows arterial fibrinoid necrosis, intimal and medial proliferation (onion skinning), severe luminal narrowing, and thrombosis. A retrospective multicenter study of 91 patients and 427 controls showed that patients treated with corticosteroids were more likely to develop scleroderma renal crisis.[49] Risk factors include diffuse skin involvement, cyclosporine use, glucocorticoid use, cyclosporine, autoantibodies, heart failure, and pericardial effusion.[50] One of the largest cohorts with 1068 patients of scleroderma from 1972 to 1987 found 108 with a developing scleroderma renal crisis. Fifty percent of that group received captopril or enalapril. There was no statistical difference between the groups. The patients who did not receive ACE inhibitors had a 1-year survival of only 15% and a 5-year survival of 10%. In marked contrast, patients treated with ACE inhibitors had an impressive 1-year survival of 76% and a 5-year survival of 65%.[51] Early initiation of ACE inhibitor significantly improved survival outcomes. The mostly studied ACE inhibitor was captopril.[3,52,53]

Pheochromocytoma

Pheochromocytoma is a rare but potentially lethal condition. Catecholamine-secreting tumors create a hyperadrenergic state, characterized by palpitations, headache, anxiety, sweating and episodic or sustained hypertension. Hypertension can present as a hypertensive emergency. If there is high clinical suspicion, treatment with alpha-blockers like phenoxybenzamine or phentolamine should be initiated before introducing a beta-blocker.[10,34]

Notable Drugs

Drugs that inhibit the vascular endothelial growth factor pathway have been approved for use in several malignancies. Its increased use has showed an increase incidence in proteinuria and hypertension, which can be severe. Hypertensive encephalopathy has been described.[54] Twenty-five percent of the patients prescribed bevacizumab and sunitinib have developed hypertension. There is some evidence the renin angiotensin system blockade and a low sodium diet was helpful in controlling blood pressure.[55]

Cocaine is a potent sympathomimetic and overdose can lead to a hypertensive emergency, not dissimilar from pheochromocytoma-induced paroxysmal hypertension. Cocaine is sometimes adulterated with fentanyl or other substances. Initial therapy can be given using intravenous nitroprusside, nitroglycerin, or calcium channel blockers.

REFERENCES

1. Whelton PK, Carey RM, Aronow WS, et al. 2017 ACC/AHA/AAPA/ABC/ACPM/AGS/APhA/ASH/ASPC/NMA/PCNa guideline for the prevention, detection, evaluation, and management of high blood pressure in adults: a report of the American College of Cardiology/American Heart Association Task Force on Clinical Practice Guidelines. Hypertension 2018; 71(6):e13–115.
2. Taylor DA. Hypertensive crisis: a review of pathophysiology and treatment. Crit Care Nurs Clin North Am 2015;27(4):439–47.
3. Brenner BM, Rector FC. Brenner & Rector's the kidney. 10th edition. Philadelphia: Saunders Elsevier; 2016.
4. Burt VL, Whelton P, Roccella EJ, et al. Prevalence of hypertension in the us adult population. results from the third National Health and Nutrition Examination Survey, 1988-1991. Hypertension 1995;25(3): 305–13.
5. Salkic S, Batic-Mujanovic O, Ljuca F, et al. Clinical presentation of hypertensive crises in emergency medical services. Mater Sociomed 2014;26(1): 12–6.
6. Shah M, Patil S, Patel B, et al. Trends in hospitalization for hypertensive emergency, and relationship of end-organ damage with in-hospital mortality. Am J Hypertens 2017;30(7):700–6.
7. Kotchen TA. Historical trends and milestones in hypertension research: a model of the process of translational research. Hypertension 2011;58(4): 522–38.
8. Brunner HR, Laragh JH, Baer L, et al. Essential hypertension: renin and aldosterone, heart attack and stroke. N Engl J Med 1972;286(9):441–9.
9. Meininger GA, Davis MJ. Cellular mechanisms involved in the vascular myogenic response. Am J Physiol 1992;263(3 Pt 2):H647–59.
10. Longo DL, Harrison TR. Harrison's principles of internal medicine. 18th edition. New York: McGraw-Hill; 2012.
11. Wallach R, Karp RB, Reves JG, et al. Pathogenesis of paroxysmal hypertension developing during and after coronary bypass surgery: a study of hemodynamic and humoral factors. Am J Cardiol 1980; 46(4):559–65.
12. Ault MJ, Ellrodt AG. Pathophysiological events leading to the end-organ effects of acute hypertension. Am J Emerg Med 1985;3(6 Suppl):10–5.
13. Granger JP, Alexander BT, Llinas M. Mechanisms of pressure natriuresis. Curr Hypertens Rep 2002;4(2): 152–9.
14. Wallbach M, Lach N, Stock J, et al. Direct assessment of adherence and drug interactions in patients with hypertensive crisis-A cross-sectional study in the Emergency Department. J Clin Hypertens (Greenwich) 2018. https://doi.org/10.1111/jch. 13448.
15. Saguner AM, Dur S, Perrig M, et al. Risk factors promoting hypertensive crises: evidence from a longitudinal study. Am J Hypertens 2010;23(7):775–80.
16. Mozaffarian D, Benjamin EJ, Go AS, et al. Heart disease and stroke statistics-2016 update: a report

from the American heart association. Circulation 2016;133(4):e38–360.

17. Amraoui F, Van Der Hoeven NV, Van Valkengoed IG, et al. Mortality and cardiovascular risk in patients with a history of malignant hypertension: a case-control study. J Clin Hypertens (Greenwich) 2014; 16(2):122–6.

18. Andrade DO, Santos SPO, Pinhel MAS, et al. Effects of acute blood pressure elevation on biochemical-metabolic parameters in individuals with hypertensive crisis. Clin Exp Hypertens 2017;39(6):553–61.

19. Prisant LM, Carr AA, Hawkins DW. Treating hypertensive emergencies: controlled reduction of blood pressure and protection of target organs. Postgrad Med 1993;93(2):92–110.

20. Varon J, Marik PE. Clinical review: the management of hypertensive crises. Crit Care 2003;7(5):374–84.

21. Powers WJ, Rabinstein AA, Ackerson T, et al. 2018 Guidelines for the early management of patients with acute ischemic stroke: a guideline for healthcare professionals from the American heart association/American stroke association. Stroke 2018;49(3): e46–110.

22. Varon JJD. Treatment of acute severe hypertension 2008;68(3):283–97.

23. Benjamin EJ, Virani SS, Callaway CW, et al. Heart disease and stroke statistics—2018 update: a report from the American Heart Association. Circulation 2018;137(12):e67–492.

24. Hemphill JC 3rd, Greenberg SM, Anderson CS, et al. Guidelines for the management of spontaneous intracerebral hemorrhage: a guideline for healthcare professionals from the American heart association/American stroke association. Stroke 2015;46(7):2032–60.

25. Anderson CS, Selim MH, Molina CA, et al. Intensive blood pressure lowering in intracerebral hemorrhage. Stroke 2017;48(7):2034–7.

26. Moullaali TJ, Wang X, Martin RH, et al. Statistical analysis plan for pooled individual patient data from two landmark randomized trials (INTERACT2 and ATACH-II) of intensive blood pressure lowering treatment in acute intracerebral hemorrhage. Int J Stroke 2018. https://doi.org/10.1177/1747493018813695.

27. Mulè G, Sorce A, Giambrone M, et al. The unsolved conundrum of optimal blood pressure target during acute haemorrhagic stroke: a comprehensive analysis. High Blood Press Cardiovasc Prev 2019. https://doi.org/10.1007/s40292-019-00305-9.

28. Arnoldus EP, Van Laar T. A reversible posterior leukoencephalopathy syndrome. N Engl J Med 1996; 334(26):1745 [author reply: 46].

29. Ekart R, Hojs R, Bevc S, et al. Asymptomatic atherosclerosis and hypertension in nondiabetic patients with chronic kidney disease. Artif Organs 2008; 32(3):220–5.

30. Varounis C, Katsi V, Nihoyannopoulos P, et al. Cardiovascular hypertensive crisis: recent evidence and review of the literature. Front Cardiovasc Med 2016;3:51.

31. Al Bannay R, Bohm M, Husain A. Heart rate differentiates urgency and emergency in hypertensive crisis. Clin Res Cardiol 2013;102(8):593–8.

32. Malachias MVB, Barbosa ECD, Martim JF, et al. 7th Brazilian guideline of arterial hypertension: chapter 14 - hypertensive crisis. Arq Bras Cardiol 2016; 107(3 Suppl 3):79–83.

33. Li JZ, Eagle KA, Vaishnava P. Hypertensive and acute aortic syndromes. Cardiol Clin 2013;31(4): 493–501, vii.

34. Larouche V, Garfield N, Mitmaker E. Extreme and cyclical blood pressure elevation in a pheochromocytoma hypertensive crisis. Case Rep Endocrinol 2018;2018:4073536.

35. Khan IA, Nair CK. Clinical, diagnostic, and management perspectives of aortic dissection. Chest 2002; 122(1):311–28.

36. Aronson S, Dyke CM, Stierer KA, et al. The ECLIPSE trials: comparative studies of clevidipine to nitroglycerin, sodium nitroprusside, and nicardipine for acute hypertension treatment in cardiac surgery patients. Anesth Analg 2008;107(4):1110–21.

37. Varon J. The diagnosis and treatment of hypertensive crises. Postgrad Med 2009;121(1):5–13.

38. Mahe I, Chassany O, Grenard AS, et al. Defining the role of calcium channel antagonists in heart failure due to systolic dysfunction. Am J Cardiovasc Drugs 2003;3(1):33–41.

39. Freda BJ, Knee AB, Braden GL, et al. Effect of transient and sustained acute kidney injury on readmissions in acute decompensated heart failure. Am J Cardiol 2017;119(11):1809–14.

40. Wan SH, Slusser JP, Hodge DO, et al. The vascular-renal connection in patients hospitalized with hypertensive crisis: a population-based study. Mayo Clin Proc Innov Qual Outcomes 2018;2(2): 148–54.

41. Nonaka K, Ubara Y, Sumida K, et al. Clinical and pathological evaluation of hypertensive emergency-related nephropathy. Intern Med 2013; 52(1):45–53.

42. Judd E, Calhoun DA. Management of hypertension in CKD: beyond the guidelines. Adv Chronic Kidney Dis 2015;22(2):116–22.

43. Lao D, Parasher PS, Cho KC, et al. Atherosclerotic renal artery stenosis–diagnosis and treatment. Mayo Clin Proc 2011;86(7):649–57.

44. Cogan JJ, Humphreys MH, Carlson CJ, et al. Renal effects of nitroprusside and hydralazine in patients with congestive heart failure. Circulation 1980; 61(2):316–23.

45. Tumlin JA, Dunbar LM, Oparil S, et al. Fenoldopam, a dopamine agonist, for hypertensive emergency: a

multicenter randomized trial. Fenoldopam Study Group. Acad Emerg Med 2000;7(6):653–62.

46. Peacock WFT, Hilleman DE, Levy PD, et al. A systematic review of nicardipine vs labetalol for the management of hypertensive crises. Am J Emerg Med 2012;30(6):981–93.

47. Cannon CM, Levy P, Baumann BM, et al. Intravenous nicardipine and labetalol use in hypertensive patients with signs or symptoms suggestive of end-organ damage in the emergency department: a subgroup analysis of the CLUE trial. BMJ Open 2013;3(3). https://doi.org/10.1136/bmjopen-2012-002338.

48. Hall VA, Guest JM. Sodium nitroprusside-induced cyanide intoxication and prevention with sodium thiosulfate prophylaxis. Am J Crit Care 1992;1(2):19–25 [quiz: 26–7].

49. Guillevin L, Berezne A, Seror R, et al. Scleroderma renal crisis: a retrospective multicentre study on 91 patients and 427 controls. Rheumatology (Oxford) 2012;51(3):460–7.

50. Gordon SM, Stitt RS, Nee R, et al. Risk factors for future scleroderma renal crisis at systemic sclerosis diagnosis. J Rheumatol 2019;46(1):85–92.

51. Steen VD, Costantino JP, Shapiro AP, et al. Outcome of renal crisis in systemic sclerosis: relation to availability of angiotensin converting enzyme (ACE) inhibitors. Ann Intern Med 1990;113(5):352–7.

52. Beckett VL, Donadio JV, Brennan LA, et al. Use of captopril as early therapy for renal scleroderma: a prospective study. Mayo Clin Proc 1985;60(11):763–71.

53. Steen VD, Medsger TA. Long-term outcomes of scleroderma renal crisis. Ann Intern Med 2000;133(8):600–3.

54. Escalante CP, Zalpour A. Vascular endothelial growth factor inhibitor-induced hypertension: basics for primary care providers. Cardiol Res Pract 2011;2011:816897.

55. Pandey AK, Singhi EK, Arroyo JP, et al. Mechanisms of VEGF (vascular endothelial growth factor) inhibitor-associated hypertension and vascular disease. Hypertension 2018;71(2):e1–8.

Contrast Nephropathy Associated with Percutaneous Coronary Angiography and Intervention

James E. Novak, MD, PhD, FNKF[a],*, Richa Handa, MD[b]

KEYWORDS

- Contrast nephropathy • Contrast-associated acute kidney injury • Coronary angiography
- Percutaneous coronary intervention

KEY POINTS

- Contrast nephropathy (CN) is acute kidney injury (AKI) that occurs within 24 to 72 hours of iodinated contrast medium (ICM) administration.
- Mechanisms of CN include hyperviscosity, free radical formation, and renal medullary oxygen supply/demand mismatch.
- Although risk factors for CN have been identified, it remains uncertain whether ICM causes or is simply associated with AKI.
- The cornerstones of CN prevention are using low-osmolal ICM, intravenous hydration, and statins, especially in patients with chronic kidney disease.
- With appropriate CN risk mitigation, coronary angiography and intervention should not be routinely withheld from patients with acute coronary syndromes.

INTRODUCTION

Contrast nephropathy (CN) was first reported in 1954 as a case of anuric acute kidney injury (AKI) following intravenous (IV) pyelography.[1] In the intervening decades, CN has become "one of medicine's hobgoblins," frightening but vague, warded against by "elixirs of N-acetylcysteine (NAC) concomitantly with saline or bicarbonate."[2] Mechanistically, there are many reasons why iodinated contrast medium (ICM) could cause kidney damage; nonetheless, in clinical medicine, the existence of CN has been legitimately questioned. In patients with acute coronary syndromes (ACS), percutaneous coronary intervention (PCI) has been withheld frequently for fear of CN. In this review, the authors discuss the experimental and clinical evidence for and against CN, risk factors and clinical outcomes, and preventive strategies.

CONTRAST NEPHROPATHY NOMENCLATURE AND DEFINITIONS

AKI associated with administration of ICM has been variably referred to as contrast-induced nephropathy, radiocontrast-induced nephropathy, contrast-induced AKI, contrast-associated AKI, contrast material–induced nephrotoxicity, contrast dye nephropathy, or simply contrast nephropathy, which is the term used in this review.[3] Disease

Disclosure Statement: Neither J.E. Novak nor R. Handa report any relevant financial disclosures or conflicts of interest.
[a] Division of Nephrology, Henry Ford Hospital, Wayne State University, CFP-505, 2799 West Grand Boulevard, Detroit, MI 48202, USA; [b] Division of Nephrology, Henry Ford Hospital, CFP-506, 2799 West Grand Boulevard, Detroit, MI 48202, USA
* Corresponding author.
E-mail address: jnovak2@hfhs.org

Cardiol Clin 37 (2019) 287–296
https://doi.org/10.1016/j.ccl.2019.04.004

associated with gadolinium-based contrast agents is not discussed here.

Historically, CN has been defined as a serum creatinine (SCr) increase of 0.5 to 1 mg/dL or 25% to 100% within 24 to 72 hours of ICM administration, often transient, with improvement back to baseline within 4 to 7 days.[4] More recently, the definition of AKI has been standardized by criteria of Risk, Injury, Failure, Loss, and End-Stage Renal Disease (RIFLE); the Acute Kidney Injury Network (AKIN); and the Kidney Disease Improving Global Outcomes (KDIGO) foundation. Diagnosis of AKI by the preferred KDIGO criteria requires, at a minimum, that SCr increase by 0.3 mg/dL within 48 hours or 50% within 7 days or that urine output decrease to less than 0.5 mL/kg per hour for 6 hours.[5–7]

MECHANISMS OF INJURY

One of the ways in which ICM is thought to cause damage is based on its rheological properties, or the ways in which it affects blood flow. Early formulations of ICM were markedly hyperosmolal (1500 to >2000 mOsm/kg; **Table 1**). Hyperosmolal ICM may cause erythrocyte dehydration and rigidity, producing tightly packed, highly viscous erythrocyte microthrombi.[8,9]

Hyperviscosity of blood and urine may be more critical than hyperosmolality in the pathogenesis of CN. By the Poiseuille law, resistance (R) to fluid flow is proportional to viscosity (η):[10]

$$R \propto \eta$$

Thus, highly viscous ICM increases resistance, both to blood flow in the renal vasculature as well as to urine flow in the renal tubules, as manifested by a persistent nephrogram on fluoroscopy.[11] Moreover, fluid flow (Q) is directly proportional to the fourth power of the vessel radius (r) and inversely proportional to the vessel length (L) and the fluid viscosity:

$$Q \propto r^4 / (l \times \eta)$$

These relationships imply that the renal medullary vasa recta, which are long and thin (also constricted; see later in this article), are uniquely susceptible to blood sludging, or even stasis, in the presence of hyperviscosity and erythrocyte microthrombi.[10]

Synergistically, ICM promotes inflammation and vasoconstriction in this susceptible renal medullary vascular bed. ICM causes the production of reactive oxygen species, including hydroxyl, peroxide, and superoxide radicals that damage the endothelium and generate procoagulant von Willebrand factor and proinflammatory nuclear factor-κB.[12] Nitric oxide, a potent vasodilator and anti-inflammatory molecule, is scavenged by these reactive oxygen species and converted to the toxic peroxynitrite radical; conversely, production of the vasoconstrictors adenosine and endothelin-1 is stimulated. The end result of these changes is intense vasoconstriction, inflammation, clotting, and endothelial damage.

This combination of rheological and oxidative damage causes an oxygen supply/demand mismatch in the renal medulla. Oxygen tension is especially low (20 mm Hg) in the renal medulla at baseline, and ICM can further compromise oxygen delivery to this region by 40% to 60%.[9,10] Concomitantly, oxygen consumption increases as the osmotic diuresis caused by ICM accelerates the workload of Na/K/2Cl transporters in the loop of Henle.[13,14] Hypoxia in the outer medulla has been demonstrated in rodent models of CN, and is worse with high viscosity, iso-osmolal ICM (IOCM; iotrolan) than with low-viscosity, low-osmolal ICM (LOCM; iopromide).[15] It is worth

---

Table 1
Physicochemical characteristics of common types of iodinated contrast media

Type	Examples	Molecular Weight, Da	Osmolality, mOsm/kg	Viscosity, mPa•s
HOCM ionic monomers	Diatrizoate (Hypaque)	810	1502	9.3
LOCM non-ionic monomers	Iohexol (Omnipaque)	821	667	10.9
	Iopamidol (Isovue)	777	640	8.4
IOCM non-ionic dimers	Iotrolan (Isovist)	1626	317	25.3
	Iodixanol (Visipaque)	1550	290	20.7

Osmolality data given at concentration of 300 to 320 mg iodine/mL and 37°C. Viscosity data given at 20°C.
Abbreviations: HOCM, high osmolal contrast medium; IOCM, iso-osmolal contrast medium; LOCM, low-osmolal contrast medium.
Data from Krause W, Schneider PW. Chemistry of x-ray contrast agents. In: Krause W, editor. Contrast agents II. Berlin, Heidelberg: Springer-Verlag Berlin Heidelberg; 2002.

noting that 1 molecule of dimeric IOCM is made by essentially linking 2 monomers of LOCM, so normal osmolality is bought at the expense of high viscosity in the physiologic milieu, which may be a poor bargain (see **Table 1**).[10,16]

Finally, ICM can cause cell death and dysfunction of cellular machinery. In addition to ischemic injury caused by the hypoxia described previously, ICM has been directly implicated in endothelial and tubule cell apoptosis and impaired proliferation, loss of planar cell polarity and tight junction integrity, and abnormal mitochondrial membrane potential.[10] In vitro studies with proximal tubule cells demonstrate decreased mitochondrial dehydrogenase activity with exposure to ICM, notably IOCM (iodixanol) and high-osmolal ICM (HOCM; diatrizoate).[17] Naturally, cell injury is likely augmented in the presence of other risk factors, such as hypotension and PCI-associated atheroembolism.

CLINICAL COURSE AND OUTCOMES

Although damage from ICM is thought to take place within minutes, increases in SCr lag by 1 to 2 days and frequently resolve by 4 to 7 days.[4] Urine microscopy and kidney biopsy show acute tubular necrosis, although the fractional excretion of sodium is often less than 1%. "Osmotic nephrosis," tubule cell vacuolization attributed to exposure to hyperosmolal urine, has also been described.[18] The differential diagnosis for CN includes prerenal azotemia, acute interstitial nephritis, and atheroembolism.

Even though the SCr increase may be transient, a single episode of AKI attributed to ICM is associated with a heightened risk of adverse events. In a cohort of 1160 hospitalized patients undergoing coronary angiography, CN conferred increased risks of prolonged hospitalization, dialysis initiation, and short- and long-term mortality (**Figs. 1** and **2**). Chronic kidney disease (CKD) further increased the likelihood of these adverse events.[19] Similarly, in a cohort of 696 patients with acute myocardial infarction (MI) without decreased ejection fraction or hemodynamic instability, CN was associated with increased all-cause mortality (24% with AKI vs 3.4% without AKI, $P <.001$). The incidence of CN in these high-risk populations was 15.8% to 19.0%.[20] One study of 2823 patients found that the incidence of CN ranged from 4.4% to 11.3% based on the definition used (SCr increase of 0.3 mg/dL or 25%), but that long-term mortality was worse with either of these definitions and proportional to AKI severity.[21]

In patients with ACS, PCI is reckoned to be a 2-sided coin, saving hearts at the expense of kidneys; thus, one area of intense focus has been CN risk stratification. One of the most celebrated stratification schemes is the so-called Mehran score.[22] Of 8357 patients undergoing PCI, 8 baseline and procedural characteristics were identified as multivariate predictors of CN:

1. Hypotension
2. Intra-aortic balloon pump use
3. Congestive heart failure (CHF)
4. Age older than 75 years
5. Anemia
6. Diabetes
7. ICM volume greater than 100 mL

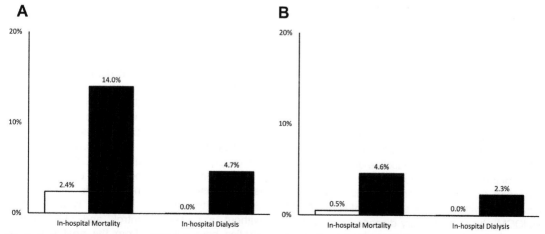

Fig. 1. In-hospital outcomes of CN following coronary angiography. (*A*) Patients with CKD and CN. (*B*) Non-CKD patients and CN. White bar, non-CN; black bar, CN. All comparisons P<.01. (*From* Neyra JA, Shah S, Mooney R, et al. Contrast-induced acute kidney injury following coronary angiography: a cohort study of hospitalized patients with or without chronic kidney disease. Nephrol Dial Transplant 2013;28(6):1467; with permission.)

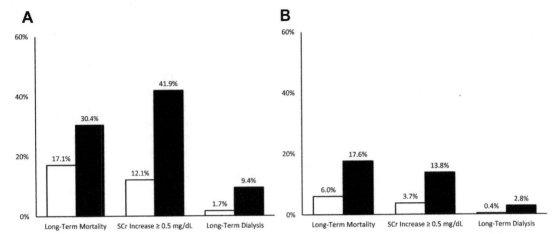

Fig. 2. Long-term outcomes of CN following coronary angiography. (*A*) Patients with CKD and CN. (*B*) Non-CKD patients and CN. White bar, non-CN; black bar, CN. All comparisons *P*<.015. (*From* Neyra JA, Shah S, Mooney R, et al. Contrast-induced acute kidney injury following coronary angiography: a cohort study of hospitalized patients with or without chronic kidney disease. Nephrol Dial Transplant 2013;28(6):1468; with permission.)

8. SCr greater than 1.5 mg/dL or estimated glomerular filtration rate (eGFR) 40 to 60, 20 to 40, or less than 20 mL/min/1.73 m^2

Each variable was assigned a point value, and the total number of points translated to a graded risk of AKI and dialysis initiation.

Recently, more risk scores have been developed to assess CN risk and many more risk factors have been documented. In a study of 963 consecutive patients, the "thrombolysis in myocardial infarction risk index" (TRI) provided a simplified risk prediction formula in patients with ST-elevation MI undergoing PCI (area under the receiver operating curve [AUC] 0.740, *P*<.001)[23]:

TRI = (heart rate × [age/10]^2) / (systolic blood pressure)

In a study of 1280 comparable patients, the "predicting bleeding complications in patients undergoing stent implantation and subsequent dual antiplatelet therapy" (PRECISE-DAPT) score, which is composed of entirely different variables such as hemoglobin, white blood cell count, and prior bleeding risk, also predicted CN (AUC 0.834, *P* = .017).[24] Additional characteristics, including hyperglycemia, baseline atrial fibrillation and diastolic dysfunction, and hypovolemia assessed by inferior vena cava diameter were associated with CN, whereas type of ICM (LOCM vs IOCM), type of coronary disease (occlusive vs nonocclusive), type of vascular access (transradial vs transfemoral), method of ICM administration (intra-arterial vs intravenous), and left ventricular end-diastolic pressure were not.[25–33]

DOES CONTRAST NEPHROPATHY EXIST?

Correlation does not imply causation, and many in the nephrology community have begun to question whether ICM actually causes AKI. Evidence in favor of CN includes, principally, the solid experimental evidence and convincing mechanistic underpinnings for ICM toxicity previously described. In clinical medicine, CN in the bygone era of HOCM may have been a distinct entity from AKI associated with more modern formulations of ICM. Although both iohexol (LOCM) and diatrizoate (HOCM) are toxic to human renal tubule cells, diatrizoate is more cytotoxic and promotes caspase-mediated apoptosis.[34] Although a meta-analysis of clinical trials did not show much difference between LOCM and HOCM in the general patient population, those with CKD had a much lower risk of SCr increase greater than 0.5 mg/dL with LOCM versus HOCM (odds ratio [OR] 0.5; 95% confidence interval [CI], 0.36–0.68).[35] Indeed, a common theme from basic science and clinical investigations is that high-risk patients (CKD, diabetes, albuminuria, advanced age, hemodynamic instability, emergency procedures) who receive high-risk ICM (HOCM, large volumes) seem to be, unsurprisingly, at high risk of CN.[36]

On the other hand, most clinical evidence of CN is circumstantial. Clinical trials have been designed to compare different types of ICM without a placebo control, and observational studies have suffered from the post hoc, ergo propter hoc ("after this, therefore because of this") logical fallacy.[37] One of the seminal proof-of-concept studies refuting the idea of CN examined the natural variation in SCr in 32,161 hospitalized patients who had at least 5 consecutive SCr determinations but who had not received ICM. The investigators found that more than half of these contrast-naïve patients showed an SCr increase of $\geq$25% and more than two-fifths showed an SCr increase of $\geq$0.4 mg/dL, which changes in SCr would have been diagnosed as CN if ICM had been administered. Moreover, the frequency of these increases was essentially the same as incidence rates of CN previously published. The investigators concluded that SCr increases tended to occur in hospitalized patients regardless of ICM administration.[38] Subsequently, similar analyses, including comparisons of patients receiving or not receiving ICM using propensity scores, gave equivalent conclusions.[37,39–41]

Is it possible that hospitalized patients with serious comorbidities are at high risk for AKI irrespective of ICM exposure? The distinction between causation and association is critical, as fear of CN may result in withholding important procedures from high-risk patients and, at worst, therapeutic nihilism or "renalism." In one study, patients with CKD were less likely than those without CKD to undergo PCI following acute MI (25.2% vs 46.8%, respectively; P<.0001), even though similar proportions of both groups should have undergone angiography based on published guidelines.[42] Unfortunately, there are no randomized, placebo-controlled trials (RCTs) to directly address the nephrotoxic potential of ICM. Although such a trial was initiated to investigate the safety of iodixanol in patients with CKD, it was regrettably terminated due to insufficient recruitment (ClinicalTrials.gov NCT03119662).[43]

CONTRAST NEPHROPATHY PREVENTION

The only known cure for CN is the tincture of time, but several strategies for prevention seem effective. These include, prominently, IV hydration to optimize volume status and kidney perfusion, as well as prescribing or withholding a number of medications or ancillary procedures.

Fluids

Volume resuscitation with IV crystalloid solutions is the foundation of CN prevention and is included in many clinical practice guidelines, but the evidence supporting this recommendation is somewhat dubious. Two recent prospective trials randomized 216 and 408 consecutive patients with ST-elevation MI undergoing PCI to 0.5 to 1 mL/kg per hour isotonic sodium chloride (NaCl) versus no fluid from procedure start to 12 to 24 hours postprocedure.[44,45] The incidence of

CN, defined as SCr increase of $\geq$25% or $\geq$0.5 mg/dL, was reduced by 35% to 48% with NaCl hydration, and was associated with less frequent in-hospital adverse events, including dialysis initiation and mortality. Conversely, a similar trial of 660 patients found that no fluid was noninferior to and more cost-effective than isotonic NaCl (CN incidence absolute difference −10%, 1-sided 95% confidence interval [CI] −2.25–2.06, 1-tailed P = .471).[46] Moreover, 5.5% of the IV NaCl group developed symptomatic heart failure with volume expansion. A meta-analysis of the available literature identified only 7 trials of 2851 patients randomized to prophylactic hydration versus no hydration.[47] Overall, IV hydration decreased the risk of CN (relative risk [RR], 0.66; 95% CI 0.55–0.79) and all-cause mortality (RR 0.57, 95% CI 0.33–0.98) but not dialysis initiation (RR 0.39, 95% CI 0.12–1.23). Importantly, prophylactic hydration conferred no advantage in patients with baseline eGFR 30 to 60 mL/min per 1.73 m^2.

In 2004, a small study generated considerable excitement for the medicinal powers of IV sodium bicarbonate ($NaHCO_3$). A total of 119 patients were randomized to receive isotonic $NaHCO_3$ versus NaCl before and after iopamidol administration, with subsequent CN rates of 1.7% and 13.6%, respectively (P = .02). The investigators proposed that bicarbonate scavenged free radicals and protected the renal medulla from oxidative damage.[48] Unfortunately, follow-up trials were unable to replicate this remarkable benefit. One meta-analysis of 20 RCTs (4280 patients) showed that IV $NaHCO_3$ outperformed IV NaCl in decreasing the frequency of CN (OR 0.67, P = .027), but not dialysis initiation or mortality, in patients with CKD, whereas a concurrent meta-analysis of 22 RCTs (5686 patients) showed no impact of fluid choice on any adverse event.[49,50] Recently, the highly publicized Prevention of Serious Adverse Events Following Angiography (PRESERVE) trial, in which 5177 patients with CKD and/or diabetes were randomized 2:2 to IV $NaHCO_3$ versus NaCl and NAC versus placebo before nonemergent angiography, showed no incremental advantage of IV $NaHCO_3$.[51]

Is oral (PO) hydration as effective as IV hydration? One trial randomized 130 low-risk patients to IV $NaHCO_3$, PO sodium citrate, or nonspecific hydration before ICM administration, and found no difference in the rate of CN.[52] A second trial randomized 225 relatively high-risk patients undergoing coronary angiography to isotonic NaCl versus PO hydration, and again found no difference in the rate of CN (6.9% vs 7.3%, P = .89); significantly, kidney function in these patients was essentially normal.[53] Finally, a pairwise

(538 patients) and network (1754 patients) meta-analysis showed no difference in the effectiveness of PO versus IV hydration, although again, patients with eGFR less than 30 mL/min per 1.73 m^2 were excluded.[54]

In summary, IV hydration seems to decrease the risk of CN in high-risk patients undergoing PCI. PO and IV hydration may give comparable protection, but the value of PO fluid has not been proven in patients with CKD. $NaHCO_3$ and NaCl also seem to give equivalent protection with regard to clinically significant outcomes. Of note, IV fluid administration guided by central venous pressure monitoring seems to be safe and effective in patients with both CKD and CHF.[55]

Medications

Following a number of inconclusive studies with simvastatin and atorvastatin, 2 seminal RCTs published in 2014 found that rosuvastatin prevented PCI-associated CN. The Statin Contrast-Induced Nephropathy Prevention (PRATO-ACS) trial randomized 504 patients with non-ST elevation ACS to rosuvastatin 20 to 40 mg daily versus placebo and showed decreased rates of CN (OR 0.38, $P = .003$) and adverse events, including 6-month mortality, with active therapy.[56] The larger Rosuvastatin Prevents Contrast-Induced Acute Kidney Injury in Patients with Diabetes (TRACK-D) trial randomized 2998 patients with type 2 diabetes and CKD undergoing coronary or peripheral angiography to rosuvastatin 10 mg daily versus placebo and also showed decreased rates of CN (2.3% vs 3.9%, respectively, $P = .01$) and heart failure with statin treatment.[57] Subsequently, several meta-analyses have shown consistent and equivalent benefits with atorvastatin and rosuvastatin for CN prophylaxis.[58–60]

In 2000, the first RCT investigating the antioxidant NAC in CN prevention was published.[61] Since then, innumerable clinical trials and meta-analyses with variable protocols and endpoints have produced contradictory findings about the benefits of NAC. In keeping with this confusion, a recent network meta-analysis of 107 RCTs including 21,450 patients undergoing coronary angiography determined that, compared with IV fluids alone, a cocktail of IV fluids, statins, and NAC decreased the risk of CN (RR 0.84, 95% CI 0.71–0.98), and that IV fluids with NAC decreased short-term mortality (RR 0.62, 95% CI 0.40–0.96).[62] Conversely, the large PRESERVE trial (see previously), published after this meta-analysis, failed to show any value of NAC.[51] Recent guidelines give a low-grade recommendation to use NAC for CN prophylaxis (see later in this article).[63]

Recently, a number of new potential medications have been proposed as CN preventives, including allopurinol, prostaglandin E1, coenzyme Q10, trimetazidine, nitrates, and oxygen.[64–66] These treatments require further study before their true value is known. Conversely, loop diuretics and nonsteroidal anti-inflammatory drugs are not recommended during ICM administration, and initiating or continuing renin-angiotensin-aldosterone inhibitors is controversial.[67,68]

Procedures

Besides medications, several therapeutic procedures have been tested for CN prevention. Historically, the first of these was periprocedural extracorporeal blood purification (EBP), intended to remove the toxic ICM from the bloodstream before kidney damage occurs. A controversial trial from 2003 randomized 114 consecutive patients with CKD (creatinine >2 mg/dL) undergoing coronary angiography to periprocedural continuous venovenous hemofiltration (CVVH) versus IV NaCl, and demonstrated reduced rates of CN, in-hospital events, and short-term and long-term mortality with CVVH.[69] This trial was criticized because (1) SCr, the biomarker of AKI, is itself removed during CVVH, possibly decreasing SCr "cosmetically" without actually preserving kidney function; (2) the CVVH group also received intensive care and anticoagulation, thus clouding the interpretation of which of several interventions was beneficial; and (3) intensive care unit transfer and CVVH for all patients at high risk of CN would be impractical and would delay life-saving PCI.[70,71] A subsequent meta-analysis of 8 trials assessing the value of hemodialysis, hemofiltration, or hemodiafiltration concluded that periprocedural EBP did not decrease the incidence of CN.[72]

Lately, interest has focused on fluid administration with matched, or isovolumetric, diuresis. Theoretically, accelerated transit of ICM through the nephron would minimize toxicity. The Renal-Guard System is a device that delivers IV NaCl in the same quantity as the urine produced during furosemide-mediated diuresis. RCTs published from 2011 to 2012 enrolled 170 to 294 high-risk patients undergoing coronary angiography to furosemide with matched IV hydration versus standard IV hydration, with decreased risk of CN in the active therapy group.[73,74] In these trials, the primary endpoint of CN was defined as an SCr increase of ≥0.3 to 0.5 mg/dL or ≥25% within 48 hours of ICM exposure, the latter of which would not qualify as AKI by currently accepted KDIGO criteria.[7] In addition, in one of these trials, the furosemide with matched hydration group received 62% more fluid volume than the standard hydration group, making it difficult to attribute the benefit to the active therapy alone.[73] A subsequent meta-analysis of 4 trials including 698 patients concluded that furosemide with matched hydration versus standard IV hydration decreased the risk of CN (OR 0.31, 95% CI 0.19–0.50).[75] Larger RCTs are under way to further explore the role of this approach in CN prophylaxis.

Remote ischemic preconditioning or postconditioning (RIPC) has also captured the imagination as a medical correlate of Einstein's "spooky action at a distance." One RCT randomized 225 patients with non-ST elevation MI undergoing PCI to IV hydration with or without 4 cycles of 1-minute inflation/deflation of the angiography balloon during PCI.[76] The patients who received the inflation/deflation cycles had a markedly decreased risk of CN (OR 0.34, 95% CI 0.16–0.71), a benefit attributed to neurohumoral mediators released during mechanical stress. These findings have been replicated in some but not all subsequent studies, although protocols differed.[77,78] The role of RIPC in preventing CN is currently undetermined.

Guidelines

The KDIGO 2012 Clinical Practice Guideline makes several recommendations regarding prevention of CN. These include using the lowest possible volume of LOCM or IOCM and periprocedural hydration with IV NaCl or NaHCO$_3$, with a suggestion to use NAC but not theophylline, fenoldopam, or EBP.[63] The 2018 update to the European Society of Urogenital Radiology Contrast Medium Safety Committee guidelines echoes these endorsements, excepting the use of NAC, and adds that the risk of AKI caused by ICM has been overstated.[79,80]

SUMMARY

Although experimental data reinforce the notion that ICM may cause kidney damage by rheological, oxidative, and hemodynamic mechanisms, clinical evidence for CN is plagued by inconsistent definitions and attribution errors. Patients at high risk for cardiovascular events and mortality are also, unsurprisingly, at high risk for AKI. Unfortunately, unwarranted fear of CN leads to therapeutic nihilism: withholding life-saving PCI from those who would benefit. The most prudent course seems to be evidence-based risk management and prophylaxis, with less toxic ICM and adequate IV hydration in patients with CKD, to avoid CN after coronary angiography or PCI.

REFERENCES

1. Bartels ED, Brun GC, Gammeltoft A, et al. Acute anuria following intravenous pyelography in a patient with myelomatosis. Acta Med Scand 1954; 150:297–302.
2. Wagner B. Scared to the marrow: pitfalls and pearls in renal imaging. Adv Chronic Kidney Dis 2017;24: 136–7.
3. Harjai KJ, Raizada A, Shenoy C, et al. A comparison of contemporary definitions of contrast nephropathy in patients undergoing percutaneous coronary intervention and a proposal for a novel nephropathy grading system. Am J Cardiol 2008;101:812–9.
4. Esson ML, Schrier RW. Diagnosis and treatment of acute tubular necrosis. Ann Intern Med 2002;137: 744–52.
5. Bellomo R, Ronco C, Kellum JA, et al, Acute Dialysis Quality Initiative workgroup. Acute renal failure - definition, outcome measures, animal models, fluid therapy and information technology needs: the Second International Consensus Conference of the Acute Dialysis Quality Initiative (ADQI) Group. Crit Care 2004;8:R204–12.
6. Mehta RL, Kellum JA, Shah SV, et al. Acute Kidney Injury Network: report of an initiative to improve outcomes in acute kidney injury. Crit Care 2007; 11:R31.
7. Kellum JA, Lameire N, Aspelin P, et al. Kidney disease: improving global outcomes (KDIGO) acute kidney injury work group. KDIGO clinical practice guideline for acute kidney injury. Kidney Int 2012;2: 19–36.
8. Do C. Intravenous contrast: friend or foe? A review on contrast-induced nephropathy. Adv Chronic Kidney Dis 2017;24:147–9.
9. McCullough PA. Contrast-induced acute kidney injury. J Am Coll Cardiol 2008;51:1419–28.
10. Persson PB, Hansell P, Liss P. Pathophysiology of contrast medium-induced nephropathy. Kidney Int 2005;68:14–22.
11. Lenhard DC, Pietsch H, Sieber MA, et al. The osmolality of nonionic, iodinated contrast agents as an important factor for renal safety. Invest Radiol 2012;47:503–10.
12. Scoditti E, Massaro M, Montinari MR. Endothelial safety of radiological contrast media: why being concerned. Vascul Pharmacol 2013;58:48–53.
13. Brezis M, Rosen S. Hypoxia of the renal medulla—its implications for disease. N Engl J Med 1995;332: 647–55.
14. Lubbers DW, Baumgartl H. Heterogeneities and profiles of oxygen pressure in brain and kidney as examples of the pO2 distribution in the living tissue. Kidney Int 1997;51:372–80.
15. Liss P, Nygren A, Erikson U, et al. Injection of low and iso-osmolar contrast medium decreases

oxygen tension in the renal medulla. Kidney Int 1998;53:698–702.

16. Jost G, Lengsfeld P, Lenhard DC, et al. Viscosity of iodinated contrast agents during renal excretion. Eur J Radiol 2011;80:373–7.

17. Hardiek K, Katholi RE, Ramkumar V, et al. Proximal tubule cell response to radiographic contrast media. Am J Physiol Renal Physiol 2001;280:F61–70.

18. Bucher AM, De Cecco CN, Schoepf UJ, et al. Is contrast medium osmolality a causal factor for contrast-induced nephropathy? Biomed Res Int 2014;2014:931413.

19. Neyra JA, Shah S, Mooney R, et al. Contrast-induced acute kidney injury following coronary angiography: a cohort study of hospitalized patients with or without chronic kidney disease. Nephrol Dial Transplant 2013;28:1463–71.

20. Sun G, Chen P, Wang K, et al. Contrast-induced nephropathy and long-term mortality after percutaneous coronary intervention in patients with acute myocardial infarction. Angiology 2018. 3319718803677.

21. Chen SQ, Liu Y, Smyth B, et al. Clinical implications of contrast-induced nephropathy in patients without baseline renal dysfunction undergoing coronary angiography. Heart Lung Circ 2018. [Epub ahead of print].

22. Mehran R, Aymong ED, Nikolsky E, et al. A simple risk score for prediction of contrast-induced nephropathy after percutaneous coronary intervention: development and initial validation. J Am Coll Cardiol 2004;44:1393–9.

23. Kaya A, Karatas A, Kaya Y, et al. A new and simple risk predictor of contrast-induced nephropathy in patients undergoing primary percutaneous coronary intervention: TIMI risk index. Cardiol Res Pract 2018; 2018:5908215.

24. Cinar T, Tanik VO, Arugaslan E, et al. The association of PRECISE-DAPT score with development of contrast-induced nephropathy in patients with ST-elevation myocardial infarction undergoing primary percutaneous coronary intervention. Cardiovasc Interv Ther 2018. [Epub ahead of print].

25. Prasitlumkum N, Kanitsoraphan C, Kittipibul V, et al. Baseline atrial fibrillation is associated with contrast-induced nephropathy after cardiac catheterization in coronary artery disease: systemic review and meta-analysis. Clin Cardiol 2018;41(12):1555–62.

26. Qin YH, Yan GL, Ma CL, et al. Effects of hyperglycaemia and elevated glycosylated haemoglobin on contrast-induced nephropathy after coronary angiography. Exp Ther Med 2018;16:377–83.

27. Demir OM, Lombardo F, Poletti E, et al. Contrast-induced nephropathy after percutaneous coronary intervention for chronic total occlusion versus non-occlusive coronary artery disease. Am J Cardiol 2018;122(11):1837–42.

28. Barbieri L, Verdoia M, Suryapranata H, et al, Novara Atherosclerosis Study Group (NAS).. Impact of vascular access on the development of contrast induced nephropathy in patients undergoing coronary angiography and/or percutaneous coronary intervention. Int J Cardiol 2019;275:48–52.

29. Lima FV, Singh S, Parikh PB, et al. Left ventricular end diastolic pressure and contrast-induced acute kidney injury in patients with acute coronary syndrome undergoing percutaneous coronary intervention. Cardiovasc Revasc Med 2018;19:16–20.

30. Azzalini L, Vilca LM, Lombardo F, et al. Incidence of contrast-induced acute kidney injury in a large cohort of all-comers undergoing percutaneous coronary intervention: comparison of five contrast media. Int J Cardiol 2018;273:69–73.

31. Gungoren F, Besli F, Tanriverdi Z, et al. Inferior vena cava assessment can predict contrast-induced nephropathy in patients undergoing cardiac catheterization: a single-center prospective study. Echocardiography 2018;35(12):1915–21.

32. Chaudhury P, Armanyous S, Harb SC, et al. Intra-arterial versus intravenous contrast and renal injury in chronic kidney disease: a propensity-matched analysis. Nephron 2019;141(1):31–40.

33. Han B, Li Y, Dong Z, et al. Diastolic dysfunction predicts the risk of contrast-induced nephropathy and outcome post-emergency percutaneous coronary intervention in AMI patients with preserved ejection fraction. Heart Vessels 2018;33:1149–58.

34. Duan S, Zhou X, Liu F, et al. Comparative cytotoxicity of high-osmolar and low-osmolar contrast media on HKCs in vitro. J Nephrol 2006;19:717–24.

35. Barrett BJ, Carlisle EJ. Metaanalysis of the relative nephrotoxicity of high- and low-osmolality iodinated contrast media. Radiology 1993;188:171–8.

36. Pan HC, Wu XH, Wan QL, et al. Analysis of the risk factors for contrast-induced nephropathy in over-aged patients receiving coronary intervention. Exp Biol Med (Maywood) 2018;243:970–5.

37. Luk L, Steinman J, Newhouse JH. Intravenous contrast-induced nephropathy-the rise and fall of a threatening idea. Adv Chronic Kidney Dis 2017;24: 169–75.

38. Newhouse JH, Kho D, Rao QA, et al. Frequency of serum creatinine changes in the absence of iodinated contrast material: implications for studies of contrast nephrotoxicity. AJR Am J Roentgenol 2008;191:376–82.

39. McDonald RJ, McDonald JS, Bida JP, et al. Intravenous contrast material-induced nephropathy: causal or coincident phenomenon? Radiology 2013;267: 106–18.

40. McDonald JS, McDonald RJ, Comin J, et al. Frequency of acute kidney injury following intravenous contrast medium administration: a systematic review and meta-analysis. Radiology 2013;267:119–28.

41. Hinson JS, Ehmann MR, Fine DM, et al. Risk of acute kidney injury after intravenous contrast media administration. Ann Emerg Med 2017;69:577–586 e574.

42. Chertow GM, Normand SL, McNeil BJ. "Renalism": inappropriately low rates of coronary angiography in elderly individuals with renal insufficiency. J Am Soc Nephrol 2004;15:2462–8.

43. A study to explore the renal safety of visipaque injection 320 mgI/mL in patients with chronic kidney disease. ClinicalTrials.gov: U.S. National Library of Medicine; 2018.

44. Jurado-Roman A, Hernandez-Hernandez F, Garcia-Tejada J, et al. Role of hydration in contrast-induced nephropathy in patients who underwent primary percutaneous coronary intervention. Am J Cardiol 2015;115:1174–8.

45. Luo Y, Wang X, Ye Z, et al. Remedial hydration reduces the incidence of contrast-induced nephropathy and short-term adverse events in patients with ST-segment elevation myocardial infarction: a single-center, randomized trial. Intern Med 2014; 53:2265–72.

46. Nijssen EC, Rennenberg RJ, Nelemans PJ, et al. Prophylactic hydration to protect renal function from intravascular iodinated contrast material in patients at high risk of contrast-induced nephropathy (AMACING): a prospective, randomised, phase 3, controlled, open-label, non-inferiority trial. Lancet 2017;389:1312–22.

47. Jiang Y, Chen M, Zhang Y, et al. Meta-analysis of prophylactic hydration versus no hydration on contrast-induced acute kidney injury. Coron Artery Dis 2017;28:649–57.

48. Merten GJ, Burgess WP, Gray LV, et al. Prevention of contrast-induced nephropathy with sodium bicarbonate: a randomized controlled trial. JAMA 2004; 291:2328–34.

49. Zhang B, Liang L, Chen W, et al. The efficacy of sodium bicarbonate in preventing contrast-induced nephropathy in patients with pre-existing renal insufficiency: a meta-analysis. BMJ Open 2015;5: e006989.

50. Zapata-Chica CA, Bello Marquez D, Serna-Higuita LM, et al. Sodium bicarbonate versus isotonic saline solution to prevent contrast-induced nephropathy : a systematic review and meta-analysis. Colomb Med (Cali) 2015;46:90–103.

51. Weisbord SD, Gallagher M, Jneid H, et al. Outcomes after angiography with sodium bicarbonate and acetylcysteine. N Engl J Med 2018;378: 603–14.

52. Martin-Moreno PL, Varo N, Martinez-Anso E, et al. Comparison of intravenous and oral hydration in the prevention of contrast-induced acute kidney injury in low-risk patients: a randomized trial. Nephron 2015;131:51–8.

53. Akyuz S, Karaca M, Kemaloglu Oz T, et al. Efficacy of oral hydration in the prevention of contrast-induced acute kidney injury in patients undergoing coronary angiography or intervention. Nephron Clin Pract 2014;128:95–100.

54. Zhang W, Zhang J, Yang B, et al. Effectiveness of oral hydration in preventing contrast-induced acute kidney injury in patients undergoing coronary angiography or intervention: a pairwise and network meta-analysis. Coron Artery Dis 2018;29:286–93.

55. Qian G, Fu Z, Guo J, et al. Prevention of contrast-induced nephropathy by central venous pressure-guided fluid administration in chronic kidney disease and congestive heart failure patients. JACC Cardiovasc Interv 2016;9:89–96.

56. Leoncini M, Toso A, Maioli M, et al. Early high-dose rosuvastatin for contrast-induced nephropathy prevention in acute coronary syndrome: results from the PRATO-ACS Study (Protective Effect of Rosuvastatin and Antiplatelet Therapy on contrast-induced acute kidney injury and myocardial damage in patients with Acute Coronary Syndrome). J Am Coll Cardiol 2014;63:71–9.

57. Han Y, Zhu G, Han L, et al. Short-term rosuvastatin therapy for prevention of contrast-induced acute kidney injury in patients with diabetes and chronic kidney disease. J Am Coll Cardiol 2014;63:62–70.

58. Liu YH, Liu Y, Duan CY, et al. Statins for the prevention of contrast-induced nephropathy after coronary angiography/percutaneous interventions: a meta-analysis of randomized controlled trials. J Cardiovasc Pharmacol Ther 2015;20:181–92.

59. Liang M, Yang S, Fu N. Efficacy of short-term moderate or high-dose rosuvastatin in preventing contrast-induced nephropathy: a meta-analysis of 15 randomized controlled trials. Medicine (Baltimore) 2017;96:e7384.

60. Liu LY, Liu Y, Wu MY, et al. Efficacy of atorvastatin on the prevention of contrast-induced acute kidney injury: a meta-analysis. Drug Des Devel Ther 2018; 12:437–44.

61. Tepel M, van der Giet M, Schwarzfeld C, et al. Prevention of radiographic-contrast-agent-induced reductions in renal function by acetylcysteine. N Engl J Med 2000;343:180–4.

62. Ma WQ, Zhao Y, Wang Y, et al. Comparative efficacy of pharmacological interventions for contrast-induced nephropathy prevention after coronary angiography: a network meta-analysis from randomized trials. Int Urol Nephrol 2018;50:1085–95.

63. Section 4: contrast-induced AKI. Kidney Int Suppl (2011) 2012;2:69–88.

64. Chen F, Liu F, Lu J, et al. Coenzyme Q10 combined with trimetazidine in the prevention of contrast-induced nephropathy in patients with coronary heart disease complicated with renal dysfunction undergoing elective cardiac catheterization: a

randomized control study and in vivo study. Eur J Med Res 2018;23:23.

65. Ahmed K, McVeigh T, Cerneviciute R, et al. Effectiveness of contrast-associated acute kidney injury prevention methods; a systematic review and network meta-analysis. BMC Nephrol 2018;19:323.

66. Qian G, Liu CF, Guo J, et al. Prevention of contrast-induced nephropathy by adequate hydration combined with isosorbide dinitrate for patients with renal insufficiency and congestive heart failure. Clin Cardiol 2019;42(1):21-5.

67. Bove T, Belletti A, Putzu A, et al. Intermittent furosemide administration in patients with or at risk for acute kidney injury: meta-analysis of randomized trials. PLoS One 2018;13:e0196088.

68. Whiting P, Morden A, Tomlinson LA, et al. What are the risks and benefits of temporarily discontinuing medications to prevent acute kidney injury? A systematic review and meta-analysis. BMJ Open 2017;7:e012674.

69. Marenzi G, Marana I, Lauri G, et al. The prevention of radiocontrast-agent-induced nephropathy by hemofiltration. N Engl J Med 2003;349:1333-40.

70. Kancha K, Lee J, Ahmed Z. Hemofiltration and the prevention of radiocontrast-agent-induced nephropathy. N Engl J Med 2004;350:836-8 [author reply: 836-8].

71. Ferrari P, Vogt B. Hemofiltration and the prevention of radiocontrast-agent-induced nephropathy. N Engl J Med 2004;350:836-8 [author reply: 836-8].

72. Cruz DN, Perazella MA, Bellomo R, et al. Extracorporeal blood purification therapies for prevention of radiocontrast-induced nephropathy: a systematic review. Am J Kidney Dis 2006;48:361-71.

73. Briguori C, Visconti G, Focaccio A, et al. Renal insufficiency after contrast media administration trial II (REMEDIAL II): RenalGuard system in high-risk patients for contrast-induced acute kidney injury. Circulation 2011;124:1260-9.

74. Marenzi G, Ferrari C, Marana I, et al. Prevention of contrast nephropathy by furosemide with matched hydration: the MYTHOS (induced diuresis with matched hydration compared to standard hydration for contrast induced nephropathy prevention) trial. JACC Cardiovasc Interv 2012;5:90-7.

75. Putzu A, Boscolo Berto M, Belletti A, et al. Prevention of contrast-induced acute kidney injury by furosemide with matched hydration in patients undergoing interventional procedures: a systematic review and meta-analysis of randomized trials. JACC Cardiovasc Interv 2017;10:355-63.

76. Deftereos S, Giannopoulos G, Tzalamouras V, et al. Renoprotective effect of remote ischemic postconditioning by intermittent balloon inflations in patients undergoing percutaneous coronary intervention. J Am Coll Cardiol 2013;61:1949-55.

77. Elserafy AS, Okasha N, Hegazy T. Prevention of contrast induced nephropathy by ischemic preconditioning in patients undergoing percutaneous coronary angiography. Egypt Heart J 2018;70:107-11.

78. Wojciechowska M, Zarebinski M, Pawluczuk P, et al. Remote ischemic preconditioning in renal protection during elective percutaneous coronary intervention. Adv Exp Med Biol 2018;1116:19-25.

79. van der Molen AJ, Reimer P, Dekkers IA, et al. Post-contrast acute kidney injury - Part 1: definition, clinical features, incidence, role of contrast medium and risk factors : recommendations for updated ESUR Contrast Medium Safety Committee guidelines. Eur Radiol 2018;28:2845-55.

80. van der Molen AJ, Reimer P, Dekkers IA, et al. Post-contrast acute kidney injury. Part 2: risk stratification, role of hydration and other prophylactic measures, patients taking metformin and chronic dialysis patients : recommendations for updated ESUR Contrast Medium Safety Committee guidelines. Eur Radiol 2018;28:2856-69.

Acute Kidney Injury, Heart Failure, and Health Outcomes

Prakash S. Gudsoorkar, MD[a],*, Charuhas V. Thakar, MD[a,b]

KEYWORDS

- Heart failure (HF) • Acute decompensated heart failure (ADHF) • Congestive heart failure (CHF)
- Acute kidney injury (AKI) • Worsening renal function (WRF) • Acute dialysis quality initiative (ADQI)
- Cardiorenal syndrome (CRS) • Health outcomes

KEY POINTS

- Acute kidney injury in acute decompensated heart failure leads to increased readmissions regardless of being transient or sustained at the time of discharge.
- Timely identification of acute kidney injury and worsening heart failure in acute decompensated heart failure patients is of utmost importance to optimize different components of heart failure treatment.
- Acute kidney injury is a strong predictor of poor outcomes and early death in patients with pulmonary artery hypertension and acute right-sided heart failure.
- Extracorporeal ultrafiltration should not be used as an initial or alternative to diuretic therapy. It should be reserved for diuretic-resistant individuals.

INTRODUCTION

Heart failure (HF) is a significant public health problem in the United States and affects 500,000 new cases per year.[1,2] It is the leading cause of hospitalizations in older adults and contributes to significant health care costs.[3] The prevalence of symptomatic congestive HF (CHF) in the United States is estimated at 2% in those over 45 years of age with a lifetime risk of CHF estimated to be 20%. With the advancement in therapeutics, HF is considered to be a chronic systemic disease and is able to be managed in a "compensated state." Although patients infrequently present with cardiogenic shock, often they present with neurohumoral dysregulation and, owing to suboptimal therapy, leading to episodes of acute decompensation.[4] There is a constant cross-talk between heart and kidney and 1 organ dysfunction or failure results in maladaptive changes in the other. Kidney dysfunction is common in patients presenting with HF, with a prevalence ranging from 20% to 57% in patients with chronic stable HF and acute decompensated HF (ADHF).[5–8] In the context of ADHF, 18% to 40% of patients will experience new worsening renal function (WRF). Regardless of when it occurs, patients with ADHF with renal dysfunction are associated with high burden of morbidity, mortality, and health care costs.[9–13] Multiple mechanisms have been proposed to explain the poor outcomes in CHF/ ADHF with kidney insufficiency. Some of these include poor systolic function, increased renin–angiotensin–aldosterone system activation, and volume overload owing to net sodium retention.[14] Herein, the authors review some of the key

Disclosure Statement: The authors have nothing to disclose.
[a] Division of Nephrology Kidney C.A.R.E. Program, University of Cincinnati, 231 Albert Sabin Way, Cincinnati, OH 45267, USA; [b] Division of Nephrology, VA Medical Center, Cincinnati, OH, USA
* Corresponding author.
E-mail address: GUDSOOPS@ucmail.uc.edu

observations from the literature regarding the interrelationship between kidney and heart dysfunction.

CARDIORENAL SYNDROME: DEFINITION AND RISK FACTORS

Cardiorenal syndrome (CRS) has been defined as the simultaneous dysfunction of both heart and kidney, regardless of which of the 2 organs sustain the initial damage. A conceptual model of CRS and related physiologic changes was proposed by Ronco and colleagues.[15] They described CRS as complex neurohormonal processes affecting heart and kidney, whereby acute or chronic dysfunction of 1 organ may perpetuate corresponding changes to the other.[15] A consensus definition for CRS would facilitate epidemiologic studies, identify a target population, develop diagnostic and prognostic strategies, and develop management strategies. The different subtypes of CRS are shown in **Table 1**.[16]

Although, there is now a consensus on the definition of acute kidney injury (AKI), there have been several terms used to describe the natural history of kidney injury during hospitalizations for ADHF. The term WRF seems to be the most common in the cardiology literature. Most commonly, patients with WRF are classified as those who have their discharge (or last) creatinine greater than at least 0.3 mg/dL relative to their admission (or first) creatinine. It should be noted, however, that this definition excludes patients who may experience AKI on admission or experience transient elevations in creatinine that return to baseline before discharge. **Table 2** shows the various definitions used in the HF literature.[17]

Several risk factors have been associated with development of WRF. These include age,[18–20] male sex,[18] prior history of renal insufficiency,[11,18–21] diabetes mellitus,[21] a history of HF,[22] prior episode of WRF, high and low systolic blood pressure, significant decrease in systolic blood pressure, atrial fibrillation, hyponatremia,[20] diastolic dysfunction, pulmonary edema, loop diuretic (furosemide) dose, or sequential nephron blockade with combination of loop and thiazide diuretics.[23]

RIGHT VENTRICULAR DYSFUNCTION AND ACUTE KIDNEY INJURY

The CRS generally focuses on left or biventricular function, its consequences of kidney, and vice versa. There are few data on right ventricular (RV) failure and its impact on kidney and vice versa. Haddad and colleagues[24] performed a retrospective analysis of 105 patients with pulmonary artery hypertension hospitalized for RV failure (184 hospitalizations). Acute RV failure was defined by the new onset of HF that required urgent inpatient management. AKI occurred in 32% patients and 23% hospitalizations. The odds of developing AKI were higher among patients with chronic kidney disease (CKD; odds ratio [OR], 3.9; 95% confidence interval [CI]. 1.1–2.4) and elevated central venous pressure (OR, 1.8; 95% CI, 1.1–2.4 per 5 mm Hg). AKI was associated with higher 30-day mortality after hospitalization for right-sided HF (OR, 5.3; 95% CI, 2.2–13.2). Another study examined the association of RV dysfunction with AKI and AKI-associated mortality in a cohort of 1879 critically ill patients with echocardiographic ventricular measurements. Overall, 43% had severe ventricular dysfunction and ventricular dysfunction was associated with 43% higher adjusted risk of AKI (95% CI, 1.14–1.80) compared with those with normal biventricular function. Isolated left ventricular, isolated RV, and biventricular dysfunction were associated with 1.34 (95% CI, 1.00–1.77), 1.35 (95% CI, 0.90–2.10), and 1.67 (95% CI, 1.23–2.31) higher adjusted risk of AKI, respectively. An episode of AKI was associated with a 2-fold greater risk of mortality and about an 8-fold higher risk of death in those with isolated RV failure, isolated left ventricular failure, and biventricular dysfunction.[25] To summarize, the physiologic complexity underlying the CRS in the setting of right and left ventricular failure may have different hemodynamic consequences.

HEART FAILURE, ACUTE KIDNEY INJURY, AND MORTALITY

Dynamic changes in renal function are frequently observed in HF population and are of importance for the guidance of treatment. In normal aging population, the glomerular filtration rate decreases by about 0.5 to 1.0 mL/min/1.732 m^2 per year; however, the loss of glomerular filtration rate is estimated to be 1 to 4 mL/min/1.732 m^2 per year in patients with CKD.[26] Damman and colleagues[13] conducted a metaanalysis in 18,634 patients with HF to determine the association of WRF with the risk of mortality and hospitalization. WRF developed in 25% of patients and was associated with 1.6 times higher odds for mortality and 1.3 times higher odds for hospitalization. CRS 1 correlated with an approximately a 5 times increased risk of mortality after 28 days, confirmed by all AKI and well as WRF definitions and the risk of mortality doubled if renal replacement therapy was required.[27] Berra and colleagues[28] analyzed the

Table 1
CRS subtypes

CRS Type	CRS Type 1 (Acute)	CRS Type 2 (Chronic)	CRS Type 3 (Acute)	CRS Type 4 (Chronic)	CRS Type 5 (Secondary)
Primary organ	Heart	Heart	Kidney	Kidney	Systemic
Primary event	ADHF/ACS	CHD	AKI	CKD	Systemic diseases (sepsis, SLE, etc)
Criteria for primary event	ESC, AHA/ACC	ESC, AHA/ACC	RIFLE-AKIN	KDOQI	Disease specific criteria
Secondary event	AKI	CKD	ADHF/ACS	CHD	AHF, ACS, AKI, CKD, CHD
Criteria for secondary event	RIFLE-AKIN	KDOQI	ESC, AHA/ACC	ESC, AHA/ACC	ESC, AHA/ACC, RIFLE-AKIN, KDOQI
Definition	Acute worsening of heart function leading to kidney dysfunction	Chronic abnormality of heart function leading to kidney dysfunction	Acute worsening of renal function leading to heart dysfunction	Chronic kidney dysfunction leading to heart dysfunction	Systemic condition leading to simultaneous dysfunction of heart and kidney.

Abbreviations: ACS, acute coronary syndrome; AHA/ACC, American heart association/American college of cardiology; AKI, acute kidney injury; AKIN, acute kidney injury network; CHD, chronic heart disease; CKD, chronic kidney disease; ESC, European cardiology society; KDOQI, kidney disease outcome quality initiative; RIFLE, risk-injury-failure-loss-end stage.

Data from Ronco C, McCullough P, Anker SD, et al. Cardio-renal syndromes: report from the consensus conference of the acute dialysis quality initiative. Eur Heart J 2010;31(6):703–11.

Table 2
Definitions and possible courses of AKI in ADHF

Possible Course of Renal Function	Definitions Used in the HF Literature
WRF	Discharge SCr at 0.3 mg/dL or 25% of admission creatinine.
Transient AKI	AKI with SCr returning to within 10% of baseline within 72 h or before discharge.
Sustained AKI	Sustained elevation of SCr (above 10% of baseline) after meeting AKI criteria for 72 h or at discharge.
AKI on admission	Peak SCr at admission followed by a decline in SCr by 0.3 mg/dL or greater during hospitalization.
No AKI	Patients with SCr fluctuations in either direction but below the 0.3-mg/dL or 1.5-times baseline creatinine threshold.

Abbreviations: AKI, acute kidney injury; SCr, serum creatinine.

From Koyner JL, Thakar CV. Acute kidney injury and critical care nephrology. NephSap 2017;16(2):141–2; with permission.

outcomes of 646 patients hospitalized with acute HF with specific emphasis on the prognostic value of AKI and WRF. Twenty-nine percent of patients had died by 1 year after admission. AKI and WRF were found to be the most powerful determinants of death. These were the subset of patients who had higher risk of poor outcomes and warranted close follow-up.

WRF during hospitalization with HF predicts adverse outcomes and prior studies define WRF using various creatinine elevations. A prospective cohort study studied 412 patients hospitalized for HF and compared the association of spectrum WRF definitions (absolute creatinine elevations of ≥0.1 mg/dL to ≥0.5 mg/dL and 25% relative elevation from baseline) with risk of death. The relative risk of mortality at 6 months of follow-up was higher with the use of restrictive definition (≥0.4 to 0.5 mg/dL increase).[29] A similar study by Gottlieb and colleagues[11] showed that the sensitivity decreased from 92% to 65% and the specificity increased from 28% to 81% for in-hospital mortality as the cutoff point for WRF was raised from 0.1 to 0.5 mg/dL.

A study by Freda and colleagues[30] analyzed a multicenter sample from the Cerner Healthfacts database and contributed information regarding in-hospital course of AKI and its impact on readmission. AKI was defined as increase of 0.3 mg/dL or greater. Three categories of AKI were recognized, namely, transient AKI (defined in **Table 2**), sustained AKI (defined in **Table 2**), and unknown AKI (defined as those with <72 hours of stay and who did not meet criteria for transient AKI). Compared with those without AKI during hospitalization, patients with sustained AKI experienced a 1.3-fold greater risk of readmission within 30 days. Of note, patients with transient AKI also experience a higher rate of readmission.

HEART FAILURE, ACUTE KIDNEY INJURY, AND RESOURCE USE

HF is a global pandemic affecting at least 26 million people worldwide.[31] Total direct medical costs for HF management has been estimated to be $30.7 billion in 2012 and projected to increase by 127% to $69.7 billon by 2030.[32] A study performed in the 18 US hospitals found that WRF was associated with escalated health care costs in patients hospitalized with acute HF, including a mean increase by $1758 per capita hospital costs among patients with WRF.[26]

An element of health care costs is captured by the outcome of duration of hospitalization and readmissions to hospital. ADHF is associated with high rate of readmissions that leads to significant individual health as well as health care burden. Several studies have demonstrated that once HF is associated with AKI or WRF, the rate of readmission multiplies several folds. A study looked at 10,000 patients from a population based prospective HF registry from 2008 to 2012. Patients with HF were identified as high frequency cluster (90.9%; mean 2.35 ± 3.68 admissions per year) and low frequency cluster (9.1%; mean 0.5 ± 0.81 admissions per year). Frequent admitters were identified as 2 or more HF admissions in the index year (n = 2587). Despite similar rates of health care use, frequent admitters had longer length of stay (4.3 days vs 4.0 days) and higher costs (€7015 vs €2967).[33] Berra and colleagues[28] analyzed 646 consecutive patients with HF coming to the emergency department at the Geneva University hospital. The primary composite endpoint was the hazard of death or readmission from the first day of hospitalization until 365 days. At 1 year after admission, 56.6% patients had been readmitted, and patients with stage 2 or 3 WRF had an increased risk of readmission compared with stage 1 WRF.

An interesting study by Freda and colleagues[30] incorporating Cerner Healthfacts database, looked at 14,000 patients with ADHF. Three clinically relevant courses of AKI were described based on the time line and persistence of serum creatinine:

a. Transient AKI defined as those meeting AKI criteria during hospitalization and subsequently returning to within 10% of admission serum creatinine value within 72 hours of onset,
b. Sustained AKI defined as those who developed AKI during hospitalization and had at least 72 hours of hospital stay but did not have a return of serum creatinine to within 10% of admission level, and
c. Unknown duration AKI, defined as patients who were discharged before at least 72 hours of hospital stay after developing AKI and did not have sufficient time to determine the resolution status.

Analysis showed that 19.2% of the study population met the primary outcome of readmission within 30 days of discharge. The readmission rate in patients without AKI was 17.7% (95% CI, 16.4%–18.9%). Compared with patients without AKI, the adjusted rate of readmission was highest in patients with sustained AKI (22.8%; 95% CI, 20.8%–24.8%; $P < .001$), followed by 20.2% in transient AKI (95% CI, 17.5%–22.8%; $P = .05$), and 19.9% (95% CI, 17.8%–21.9%; $P = .036$) in those with unknown AKI. Patients with sustained AKI were 1.3 times more likely to get readmitted at 30 days compared with those without AKI. The authors speculate a biological relation between mild degree of AKI and cross-organ dysregulation in ADHF regardless of the transient nature of renal dysfunction. The timing of onset, course, and duration of AKI in ADHF cohort stratify risk profile and the treating physician should be mindful of the outcomes so as to plan the discharge and follow-up accordingly.[30] Thakar and colleagues,[34] based on a statewide inpatient sample, investigated whether AKI, with or without CKD, would result in repeat admissions with CHF. The analyzed data from 6535 patients discharged with primary diagnosis of HF from an administrative inpatient database. During index hospitalization, 6.5% of cases were coded for AKI, whereas 16% had CKD. Fifteen percent of patients required readmission within 30 days for repeat episodes of HF. Index mortality was 1.7% in those without AKI or CKD versus 13% and 11% in those with AKI with or without CKD, respectively ($P < .0001$). Patients with AKI experienced a 30-day HF readmission rate of 21% compared with 14% in those

without AKI ($P < .0001$). By multivariate analysis, AKI without CKD was associated with the highest risk of readmission (OR, 1.81; 95% CI, 1.35–2.39) as compared with those with neither of the 2 diagnoses. Two additional studies analyzed large patient database for HF readmissions in the setting of WRF and demonstrated that WRF during HF hospitalization was an independent risk factor for readmission.[35,36]

To summarize, the subset of patients with AKI or WRF carry the highest risk of readmissions at 30 days or up to 1 year after discharge and incur a significant health care burden. The timely identification of AKI and WRF in this special cohort of patients with HF is of utmost importance to optimize treatment and decrease readmission-related morbidity and mortality.

VOLUME OVERLOAD, DIURETICS, AND ACUTE KIDNEY INJURY IN ACUTE DECOMPENSATED HEART FAILURE

Congestion in ADHF has specific consequences on the renal pathophysiology. Venous hypertension results in decreased renal perfusion, increased kidney interstitial pressure, narrowed decreased arterial-to-venous renal pressure gradient, decreased glomerular filtration rate, maladaptive autoregulatory responses, and other characteristic neurohumoral imbalances. The higher renal pressure attenuates glomerular filtration, causes tubule collapse, and triggers tubulointerstitial fibrosis.[37,38] Herein, the authors discuss the salient trials that involved diuretic therapy in the management of ADHF. Salvador and colleagues[39] conducted a metaanalysis comparing the safety and efficacy of intravenous infusion versus intravenous bolus administration of loop diuretics in CHF. Eight trials involving 254 patients were included and showed greater urine output, less ototoxicity (hearing loss and tinnitus), and similar frequency of electrolyte disturbances in patients given continuous infusion as compared with the intermittent dosing. The data were insufficient to report and compare renal safety, survival, or other significant clinical outcomes when both the dosing regimens were compared. Diuretic Optimization Strategies Evaluation in AHF (DOSE-AHF) trial was a prospective, double blinded, placebo controlled, randomized study, which used 2×2 factorial design. The trial randomly assigned 308 patients to receive furosemide administered intravenously via either intermittent bolus every 12 hours or continuous infusion, and at either a low dose (equivalent to the patient's previous oral dose) or a high dose (2.5 times the previous

Table 3
Summary of trials on UF in HF

Study	RAPID-CHF (2005)	ULOAD (2007)	ULTADISCO (2011)	CARESS-HF (2012)	CUORE (2014)	AVOID-HF (2016)
Design	RCT	RCT	RCT	RCT	RCT	RCT
No. of patients	UF:20 PT:20	UF:100 PT:100	UF:15 PT:15	UF:94 PT:94	UF:27 PT:29	UF:110 PT:114
UF arm	Single 8 h median volume removed 3213 mL	Aquadex system. Avg. UFR 500 ml/h for 12.3 ± 12 h	PRISMA Treatment duration 46 h. UF 9.7 ± 2.9 L.	Aquadex System. UFR 200 mL/h Median duration 40 h.	Dedyca device. Mean Rx 19 ± 10 h. Max UFR 500 mL/h	Aquadex flex flow system. Avg. UFR 138 mL/h for 80 ± 53 h
PT	Standard HF care	Standard HF care	Furosemide continuous infusion	SPT (algorithm based)	Standard care	Protocol guided IV loop diuretics
Difference in kidney function UF vs PT	No significant difference	No significant difference	No significant difference	Significant increase in SCr with UF. No change with PT.	Higher SCr and BUN in PT at 6 mo. No difference between UF and PT at 1 y.	No significant difference in eGFR, BUN, and SCr up to 90 d between UF and PT.

Abbreviations: PT, pharmacologic treatment; RCT, randomized control trial; SCr, serum creatinine; SPT, stepped pharmacologic therapy; UF, ultrafiltration; UFR, UF rate.
Data from Refs.[42–47]

oral dose). The efficacy endpoint was the patients' global assessment of symptoms over the course of 72 hours and the safety endpoint was change in serum creatinine from baseline to 72 hours. WRF was defined as an increase in the serum creatinine of greater than 0.3 mg/dL at any time during the 72 hours after randomization. Hypotensive patients with systolic blood pressures of less than 90 mm Hg who required inotropes or intravenous vasodilators and those with a serum creatinine of greater than 3 mg/dL were excluded. There was no significant difference in efficacy or safety endpoints for bolus versus continuous infusion. Patients assigned to intravenous bolus therapy were more likely to require a dose increase at 48 hours; however, the total dose of furosemide over 72 hours in the bolus group was not significantly different from that in the continuous infusion group (592 vs 480 mg; $P = .06$). High-dose furosemide, compared with low-dose furosemide, produced greater net fluid loss, weight loss, and relief from dyspnea, but also more frequent transient worsening of renal function (23% vs 14%). There was no significant difference in patients' global assessment of symptoms in the high-dose group ($P = .06$) and the mean change in the serum creatinine was less than 0.1 mg/dL in both groups. To summarize, there was no significant difference in symptom relief or renal safety when loop diuretics were administered as a bolus or continuous infusion. High-dose therapy improved diuresis with a trend toward improved symptom relief but caused more renal adverse events compared with low-dose therapy.[40] An interesting post hoc analysis done by Grodin and colleagues[41] compared the decongestive properties of a stepwise pharmacologic care algorithm used in CARESS-HF trial (n = 94) and standard decongestive therapy used in DOSE-HF and ROSE-HF trial (n = 107). The stepwise pharmacologic care algorithm group had greater net fluid and weight loss without being associated with renal compromise when compared with the standard decongestive therapy group.

EXTRACORPOREAL ULTRAFILTRATION IN ACUTE DECOMPENSATED HEART FAILURE

Diuretics have remained the cornerstone of therapy for volume overload in the setting of ADHF. A significant subset of patients with HF experiences diuretic resistance. Hence, there is an unmet clinical need for alternative forms of fluid removal. Over the past 2 decades, several studies have been conducted to define the physiologic rationale for clinical benefit and safety of extracorporeal ultrafiltration as the initial mode of

decongestive therapy in the management of ADHF. **Table 3** summarizes the landmark trials conducted in the field of extracorporeal therapy for HF management.[42–47] Although the current studies support the concept of using ultrafiltration in the management of HF, long-term outcomes of this approach have not been studied. Current evidence suggests that the rate of adverse events might be higher in patients subjected to ultrafiltration therapy. Accordingly, ultrafiltration in patients hospitalized with ADHF in the setting of renal dysfunction should be reserved for patients who have been refractory to pharmacologic therapy rather than a first-line therapy (see **Table 3**).

SUMMARY

AKI in ADHF leads to increased readmissions regardless of being transient or sustained at the time of discharge. Timely identification of AKI and worsening HF in patients with ADHF is of utmost importance to optimize different components of HF treatment. AKI is a strong predictor of poor outcomes and early death in patients with pulmonary artery hypertension and acute right-sided HF. Extracorporeal ultrafiltration should not be used as an initial or alternative to diuretic therapy. It should be reserved for diuretic resistant individuals.

REFERENCES

1. Savarese G, Lund LH. Global public health burden of heart failure. Card Fail Rev 2017;3(1):7–11.
2. Benjamin EJ, Virani SS, Callaway CW, et al. Heart disease and stroke statistics-2018 update: a report from the American Heart Association. Circulation 2018;137(12):e67–492.
3. Butler J, Chirovsky D, Phatak H, et al. Renal function, health outcomes, and resource utilization in acute heart failure: a systematic review. Circ Heart Fail 2010;3(6):726–45.
4. Adams KF Jr, Fonarow GC, Emerman CL, et al. Characteristics and outcomes of patients hospitalized for heart failure in the United States: rationale, design, and preliminary observations from the first 100,000 cases in the Acute Decompensated Heart Failure National Registry (ADHERE). Am Heart J 2005;149(2):209–16.
5. Investigators S, Yusuf S, Pitt B, et al. Effect of enalapril on survival in patients with reduced left ventricular ejection fractions and congestive heart failure. N Engl J Med 1991;325(5):293–302.
6. Dries DL, Exner DV, Domanski MJ, et al. The prognostic implications of renal insufficiency in asymptomatic and symptomatic patients with left ventricular systolic dysfunction. J Am Coll Cardiol 2000;35(3):681–9.

7. Cleland JG, Carubelli V, Castiello T, et al. Renal dysfunction in acute and chronic heart failure: prevalence, incidence and prognosis. Heart Fail Rev 2012;17(2):133–49.

8. de Silva R, Nikitin NP, Witte KK, et al. Incidence of renal dysfunction over 6 months in patients with chronic heart failure due to left ventricular systolic dysfunction: contributing factors and relationship to prognosis. Eur Heart J 2006;27(5):569–81.

9. Cowie MR, Komajda M, Murray-Thomas T, et al, POSH Investigators. Prevalence and impact of worsening renal function in patients hospitalized with decompensated heart failure: results of the prospective outcomes study in heart failure (POSH). Eur Heart J 2006;27(10):1216–22.

10. Forman DE, Butler J, Wang Y, et al. Incidence, predictors at admission, and impact of worsening renal function among patients hospitalized with heart failure. J Am Coll Cardiol 2004;43(1):61–7.

11. Gottlieb SS, Abraham W, Butler J, et al. The prognostic importance of different definitions of worsening renal function in congestive heart failure. J Card Fail 2002;8(3):136–41.

12. Kociol RD, Greiner MA, Hammill BG, et al. Long-term outcomes of Medicare beneficiaries with worsening renal function during hospitalization for heart failure. Am J Cardiol 2010;105(12):1786–93.

13. Damman K, Navis G, Voors AA, et al. Worsening renal function and prognosis in heart failure: systematic review and meta-analysis. J Card Fail 2007; 13(8):599–608.

14. Chae CU, Albert CM, Glynn RJ, et al. Mild renal insufficiency and risk of congestive heart failure in men and women > or =70 years of age. Am J Cardiol 2003;92(6):682–6.

15. Ronco C, Haapio M, House AA, et al. Cardiorenal syndrome. J Am Coll Cardiol 2008;52(19): 1527–39.

16. Ronco C, McCullough P, Anker SD, et al. Cardiorenal syndromes: report from the consensus conference of the acute dialysis quality initiative. Eur Heart J 2010;31(6):703–11.

17. Koyner J, Thakar CV. Acute kidney injury and critical care nephrology. NephSap, vol. 16. American Society of Nephrology; 2017. p. 141–2.

18. Damman K, Valente MA, Voors AA, et al. Renal impairment, worsening renal function, and outcome in patients with heart failure: an updated meta-analysis. Eur Heart J 2014;35(7):455–69.

19. Voors AA, Davison BA, Felker GM, et al. Early drop in systolic blood pressure and worsening renal function in acute heart failure: renal results of pre-RELAX-AHF. Eur J Heart Fail 2011;13(9):961–7.

20. Chittineni H, Miyawaki N, Gulipelli S, et al. Risk for acute renal failure in patients hospitalized for decompensated congestive heart failure. Am J Nephrol 2007;27(1):55–62.

21. Aronson D, Burger AJ. The relationship between transient and persistent worsening renal function and mortality in patients with acute decompensated heart failure. J Card Fail 2010;16(7):541–7.

22. Tang WH, Mullens W. Cardiorenal syndrome in decompensated heart failure. Heart 2010;96(4): 255–60.

23. Jentzer JC, DeWald TA, Hernandez AF. Combination of loop diuretics with thiazide-type diuretics in heart failure. J Am Coll Cardiol 2010;56(19):1527–34.

24. Haddad F, Fuh E, Peterson T, et al. Incidence, correlates, and consequences of acute kidney injury in patients with pulmonary arterial hypertension hospitalized with acute right-side heart failure. J Card Fail 2011;17(7):533–9.

25. Chen C, Lee J, Johnson AE, et al. Right ventricular function, peripheral edema, and acute kidney injury in critical illness. Kidney Int Rep 2017;2(6):1059–65.

26. Krumholz HM, Chen YT, Vaccarino V, et al. Correlates and impact on outcomes of worsening renal function in patients > or =65 years of age with heart failure. Am J Cardiol 2000;85(9):1110–3.

27. Vandenberghe W, Gevaert S, Kellum JA, et al. Acute kidney injury in cardiorenal syndrome type 1 patients: a systematic review and meta-analysis. Cardiorenal Med 2016;6(2):116–28.

28. Berra G, Garin N, Stirnemann J, et al. Outcome in acute heart failure: prognostic value of acute kidney injury and worsening renal function. J Card Fail 2015;21(5):382–90.

29. Smith GL, Vaccarino V, Kosiborod M, et al. Worsening renal function: what is a clinically meaningful change in creatinine during hospitalization with heart failure? J Card Fail 2003;9(1):13–25.

30. Freda BJ, Knee AB, Braden GL, et al. Effect of transient and sustained acute kidney injury on readmissions in acute decompensated heart failure. Am J Cardiol 2017;119(11):1809–14.

31. Ponikowski P, Anker SD, AlHabib KF, et al. Heart failure: preventing disease and death worldwide. ESC Heart Fail 2014;1(1):4–25.

32. Jackson SL, Tong X, King RJ, et al. National burden of heart failure events in the United States, 2006 to 2014. Circ Heart Fail 2018;11(12):e004873.

33. Go YY, Sellmair R, Allen JC Jr, et al. Defining a 'frequent admitter' phenotype among patients with repeat heart failure admissions. Eur J Heart Fail 2019;21(3):311–8.

34. Thakar CV, Parikh PJ, Liu Y. Acute kidney injury (AKI) and risk of readmissions in patients with heart failure. Am J Cardiol 2012;109(10):1482–6.

35. Palmer JB, Friedman HS, Waltman Johnson K, et al. Association of persistent and transient worsening renal function with mortality risk, readmissions risk, length of stay, and costs in patients hospitalized with acute heart failure. Clinicoecon Outcomes Res 2015;7:357–67.

36. Patel UD, Greiner MA, Fonarow GC, et al. Associations between worsening renal function and 30-day outcomes among Medicare beneficiaries hospitalized with heart failure. Am Heart J 2010;160(1): 132–138 e131.

37. Braam B, Cupples WA, Joles JA, et al. Systemic arterial and venous determinants of renal hemodynamics in congestive heart failure. Heart Fail Rev 2012;17(2):161–75.

38. Maxwell MH, Breed ES, Schwartz IL. Renal venous pressure in chronic congestive heart failure. J Clin Invest 1950;29(3):342–8.

39. Salvador DR, Rey NR, Ramos GC, et al. Continuous infusion versus bolus injection of loop diuretics in congestive heart failure. Cochrane Database Syst Rev 2005;(3):CD003178.

40. Felker GM, Lee KL, Bull DA, et al. Diuretic strategies in patients with acute decompensated heart failure. N Engl J Med 2011;364(9):797–805.

41. Grodin JL, Stevens SR, de Las Fuentes L, et al. Intensification of medication therapy for cardiorenal syndrome in acute decompensated heart failure. J Card Fail 2016;22(1):26–32.

42. Bart BA, Boyle A, Bank AJ, et al. Ultrafiltration versus usual care for hospitalized patients with heart failure: the relief for acutely fluid-overloaded patients with decompensated congestive heart failure (RAPID-CHF) trial. J Am Coll Cardiol 2005;46(11):2043–6.

43. Costanzo MR, Guglin ME, Saltzberg MT, et al. Ultrafiltration versus intravenous diuretics for patients hospitalized for acute decompensated heart failure. J Am Coll Cardiol 2007;49(6):675–83.

44. Giglioli C, Landi D, Cecchi E, et al. Effects of ULTRA-filtration vs. DIureticS on clinical, biohumoral and haemodynamic variables in patients with deCOmpensated heart failure: the ULTRADISCO study. Eur J Heart Fail 2011;13(3):337–46.

45. Bart BA, Goldsmith SR, Lee KL, et al. Ultrafiltration in decompensated heart failure with cardiorenal syndrome. N Engl J Med 2012;367(24):2296–304.

46. Marenzi G, Muratori M, Cosentino ER, et al. Continuous ultrafiltration for congestive heart failure: the CUORE trial. J Card Fail 2014;20(1):9–17.

47. Costanzo MR, Negoianu D, Jaski BE, et al. Aquapheresis versus intravenous diuretics and hospitalizations for heart failure. JACC Heart Fail 2016;4(2): 95–105.

Hypertension Management in Chronic Kidney Disease and Diabetes

Lessons from the Systolic Blood Pressure Intervention Trial

George Thomas, MD, MPH

KEYWORDS

- Hypertension • Chronic kidney disease • Diabetes • Guidelines • SPRINT • ACCORD BP

KEY POINTS

- Hypertension management and blood pressure goals in patients with chronic kidney disease and diabetes.
- Systolic Blood Pressure Intervention Trial results and analysis with comparison with Action to Control Cardiovascular Risk in Diabetes Blood Pressure results, and nonpharmacologic and pharmacologic approaches to hypertension management.
- Because more medications will be needed for intensive control, side effects and tolerability of medications with polypharmacy, and potential nonadherence with increasing complexity of medication regimens, should be kept in mind.

INTRODUCTION

Hypertension is a strong independent risk factor for cardiovascular disease, with observational studies showing a strong relationship between high blood pressure (BP) and increased risk of morbidity and mortality.[1] Hypertension is common in patients with chronic kidney disease (CKD), and it can be a cause or consequence of CKD.[2] The prevalence of hypertension in patients with CKD, when defined as a BP level greater than or equal to 140/90 mm Hg, is inversely related to the estimated glomerular filtration rate (eGFR), increasing from 67% in those with eGFR greater than 60 mL/min/1.73 m^2 to 92% in those with eGFR less than 30 mL/min/1.73 m^2.[3] Patients with CKD are at higher risk for hypertension-related adverse outcomes, including cardiovascular disease,[4] and therefore, the management of hypertension is particularly important in patients with CKD.

BEFORE THE SYSTOLIC BLOOD PRESSURE INTERVENTION TRIAL

Limited data from clinical trials on BP targets have shown a benefit to lowering systolic BP to less than 150 mm Hg in the general population. Both the Systolic Hypertension in the Elderly Program (SHEP) and the Hypertension in the Very Elderly Trial (HYVET) showed cardiovascular benefit with systolic BP lower than 150 mm Hg compared with higher levels.[5,6] The Japanese Trial to Assess Optimal Systolic Blood Pressure (JATOS) and the Valsartan in Elderly Systolic Hypertension (VALISH) trial did not show benefit for systolic BP lower than 140 mm Hg (compared with <150 mm Hg), but these trials were underpowered.[7,8] Results from other trials have also indicated that BP of less than 140/90 mm Hg was associated with a lower rate of cardiovascular events compared with higher BP levels.[9]

Disclosures: The author has nothing to disclose.
Center for Blood Pressure Disorders, Department of Nephrology and Hypertension, Cleveland Clinic, Cleveland Clinic Lerner College of Medicine, 9500 Euclid Avenue, Q7 Glickman Tower, Cleveland, OH 44195, USA
E-mail address: thomasg3@ccf.org

Cardiol Clin 37 (2019) 307–317
https://doi.org/10.1016/j.ccl.2019.04.006

Although there is evidence from observational studies that inadequately controlled BP is a risk factor for progression of CKD, there is uncertainty about the degree and duration of hypertension required to produce CKD.[10] In addition, there was no definitive evidence that aggressive lowering of BP slows progression of nonproteinuric CKD. In the Modified Disease in Renal Disease (MDRD) study and the African American Study of Kidney Disease and Hypertension (AASK), intensive lowering of BP did not slow progression of CKD (although post hoc analyses suggest that, in the subset of patients with significant proteinuria, intensive lowering of BP may be beneficial to slow CKD progression).[11–14] A retrospective cohort observational modeling study showed that mortality was higher among patients with CKD treated to a systolic BP less than 120 mm Hg versus 120 to 139 mm Hg.[15]

In patients with type 2 diabetes mellitus (DM), the Action to Control Cardiovascular Risk in Diabetes Blood Pressure (ACCORD BP) trial showed that there was no benefit to lowering systolic BP to less than 120 mm Hg compared with less than 140 mm Hg for the primary composite cardiovascular outcome; however, there was a reduction in stroke events in the intensive treatment group.[16] Similarly, in a trial examining role of antiplatelet agents in patients with recurrent stroke, patients did not show significant benefit to lowering systolic BP to less than 130 mm Hg compared with less than 150 mm Hg for overall risk of a recurrent stroke, except in cases of hemorrhagic stroke outcome.[17]

Based on available evidence, the guidelines before the Systolic Blood Pressure Intervention Trial (SPRINT) trial (a randomized trial of intensive vs standard blood pressure control) recommended a BP target of less than 140/90 mm Hg in patients with CKD.[18] Although the 2014 Eighth Joint National Committee (JNC 8) panel guidelines did not specify targets in patients with proteinuria, the 2012 KDIGO (Kidney Disease: Improving Global Outcomes) guidelines recommend a BP target of less than 130/80 mm Hg in proteinuric patients (although they acknowledge that the evidence was of lower quality).[19] This lower target for patients with proteinuria was also advocated in guidelines jointly published by the American Society of Hypertension and the International Society of Hypertension.[20] SPRINT was designed to answer the following question: in patients with increased cardiovascular risk, including CKD but without diabetes or stroke, does systolic BP goal of less than 120 mm Hg reduce adverse clinical events more than the currently followed systolic BP goal of less than 140 mm Hg?

SYSTOLIC BLOOD PRESSURE INTERVENTION TRIAL DESIGN AND MAIN RESULTS

SPRINT was a randomized controlled, open-label trial, and participants in the study had to be at least 50 years old, with a systolic BP of 130 to 180 mm Hg, and had to have at least 1 cardiovascular risk, which included the following: clinical or subclinical cardiovascular disease (other than stroke), CKD defined as eGFR of 20 to less than 60 mL/min/1.73 m², Framingham risk score of 15% or more, and age 75 years or older. Major exclusion criteria included diabetes, stroke, polycystic kidney disease, CKD with eGFR less than 20 mL/min/1.73 m², and proteinuria more than 1 g/d.[21]

Participants were randomized to an intensive group (target systolic BP <120 mm Hg) or to a standard group (target systolic BP <140 mm Hg). Baseline antihypertensive medications were adjusted to achieve BP goals based on randomization assignment. Dose adjustments to medications were made based on an average of 3 seated office BP measurements after a 5-minute period of rest, taken with an automated BP monitor. There was no restriction on use of any antihypertensive medication, and this was at the discretion of individual investigators. Thiazide-type diuretics were encouraged as first-line agents (with chlorthalidone encouraged as the primary thiazide-type diuretic). Participants in the intensive group were seen monthly until a target systolic BP of less than 120 mm Hg was reached. Participants in the standard group had medications adjusted to maintain a systolic BP level of between 135 and 139 mm Hg.

The primary outcome was a composite of myocardial infarction (MI), acute coronary syndrome not resulting in MI, stroke, acute decompensated heart failure (HF), or cardiovascular mortality. Secondary outcomes included individual components of the primary composite outcome, all-cause mortality, and composite of primary outcome and all-cause mortality. Renal outcomes were also assessed, as incident albuminuria (doubling of urinary albumin-to-creatinine ratio from <10 mg/g to >10 mg/g), composite of 50% decrease in eGFR or development of end-stage renal disease (ESRD; requiring long-term dialysis or kidney transplant) in patients with baseline CKD, and 30% decrease in eGFR in those without CKD.

Between 2010 and 2013, 9361 participants were enrolled in the study, with a median follow-up of 3.2 years. There were 3333 (35.5%) women and 2802 (29.9%) black participants, 2636 (28.2%) were at least 75 years old, and 2648 (28.3%) had

CKD. The average BP difference between the 2 groups was 13.1 mm Hg, with a mean systolic BP of 121.5 mm Hg in the intensive group and 134.6 mm Hg in the standard group. The difference in systolic BP between the 2 groups was achieved at 1 year, and sustained thereafter. The mean numbers of antihypertensive medications were 2.8 and 1.8 in the intensive and standard groups, respectively. The distribution of antihypertensive medication classes was similar in the 2 groups.

The primary outcome event rate was significantly lower in the intensive group compared with standard group (1.6% per year vs 2.1% per year; hazard ratio [HR] [confidence interval (CI)] 0.75 [0.64–0.89], P<.0001). This finding was driven by a significantly lower rate of HF and cardiovascular mortality in the intensive group (1.3% per year vs 2.1% per year, P = .002 for HF; 0.8% per year vs 1.4% per year, P = .0005 for cardiovascular mortality). The effects on primary outcome and mortality were consistent across the prespecified subgroups of age (<75 years vs≥75 years), gender (female vs male), race (black vs nonblack), cardiovascular disease (presence or absence at baseline), prior CKD (presence or absence at baseline), and across BP tertiles (≤132 mm Hg, >132 to <145 mm Hg, ≥145 mm Hg). Serious adverse events, including hypotension, syncope, electrolyte abnormalities, and acute kidney injury (AKI), occurred more frequently in the intensive group.[22]

SYSTOLIC BLOOD PRESSURE INTERVENTION TRIAL AND CHRONIC KIDNEY DISEASE

Most (66%) of the SPRINT participants with CKD had a baseline eGFR greater than or equal to 45 mL/min/1.73 m^2, a low median baseline albuminuria (12.8 mg/g), and a slow chronic eGFR decline during follow-up (<0.5 mL/min/1.73 m^2/y), suggesting that the CKD participants in the SPRINT generally had mild CKD and maintained their kidney function during the trial.

In a prespecified subgroup analysis of outcomes in participants with CKD, intensive reduction in BP (aiming for systolic BP <120 mm Hg) resulted in a substantial decrease in the primary outcome and all-cause death without evidence of effect modifications by baseline CKD status.[23] There was also no difference in the main kidney outcome between the 2 randomized groups in the participants with baseline CKD. The main kidney outcome, defined as a confirmed decrease in eGFR of greater than or equal to 50% or development of ESRD, occurred in 15 participants (1.1%) in the intensive group and 16 participants (1.2%) in the

standard group (HR, 0.90; 95% CI, 0.44–1.83). These findings were consistent with the observations in subgroups defined by age, sex, race, eGFR, or albuminuria, although the numbers of events in these subgroups were too small to allow meaningful interpretations. The incidence of albuminuria was not significantly different between the randomized groups. There was no difference in overall serious adverse events and adverse events associated with hypotension, syncope, bradycardia, injurious falls, hyponatremia, hypernatremia, or orthostatic hypotension between the 2 treatment groups within the CKD subgroup. However, there were increased risks for hypokalemia, hyperkalemia, and acute renal failure in the intensive group compared with the standard group.

The 2 largest clinical trials that have addressed renal disease progression in patients with nondiabetic CKD, the MDRD and AASK, showed no overall benefit of intensive BP treatment on primary kidney outcomes. However, post hoc analyses of both studies suggested a benefit of intensive BP treatment in the subgroup with significant proteinuria.[11–14] There was no benefit of intensive BP lowering on a variety of kidney outcomes in the SPRINT participants with baseline CKD; however, there was also no adverse effect on the main kidney composite outcome. The SPRINT population differed from those in previous clinical trials in the CKD population. Patients with proteinuria greater than 1 g/d were excluded from participation. Although SPRINT enrolled a racially diverse population, participants in the MDRD study were predominantly white, whereas participation in the AASK was restricted to black people. Neither the MDRD nor AASK study targeted systolic BP as low as 120 mm Hg. The totality of the data from randomized trials to date does not provide evidence of a beneficial effect of intensive BP lowering on the progression of kidney disease in patients without significant proteinuria, but it also does not provide evidence of substantial harm.

An acute decrease in glomerular filtration rate (GFR) after BP lowering is thought to be caused by hemodynamic changes in the renal microcirculation. In SPRINT, there was an acute decline in eGFR in the intensive group after randomization. In contrast, there was a slight increase in eGFR in the standard group during the first 6 months. It is likely that the higher rate of greater than or equal to 30% decline in eGFR observed in the intensive group was related to an acute hemodynamic effect on the GFR, particularly because this difference between the 2 randomized groups disappeared after the initial 6 months of treatment.

The early termination of the SPRINT intervention might have influenced the reported outcomes in the CKD subgroup. The shorter duration of follow-up might have limited evaluation of the long-term effect of the intensive BP intervention on kidney function; this is particularly important given the acute change in eGFR in the first few months. Thus, long-term follow-up of the CKD subcohort would be important.

SYSTOLIC BLOOD PRESSURE INTERVENTION TRIAL AND ACUTE KIDNEY INJURY

AKI was defined using modified KDIGO criteria incorporating only serum creatinine concentration to assess for AKI stage (ignoring the component of urine output, which was not uniformly measured).[24] These modified KDIGO criteria include the following AKI stages and serum creatinine definitions: stage 1, increase greater than or equal to 0.3 mg/dL or increase of 1.5-fold to 2.0-fold from baseline; stage 2, increase greater than 2.0-fold to 3.0-fold from baseline; and stage 3, increase greater than 3.0-fold from baseline or greater than or equal to 4.0 mg/dL with an acute increase of 0.5 mg/dL or need for renal replacement therapy.

There were 348 events adjudicated as AKI in 288 participants (3%). Two-hundred and forty-eight (86.1%) had a single AKI event during the course of the trial, 30 (10.4%) had 2 events, 5 (1.7%) had 3 events, and 5 (1.7%) had 4 or more events. AKI events were typically mild, with stage 1 being the most common AKI stage. Based on modified KDIGO criteria, numbers of AKI events in the intensive versus standard arm by KDIGO stage were 128 (58.5%) versus 81 (62.8%) in stage 1, 42 (19.2%) versus 18 (14.0%) in stage 2, and 42 (19.2%) versus 25 (19.4%) in stage 3.

Dialysis was required infrequently by participants in the intensive (n = 8) and standard (n = 6) arms and end-stage kidney disease subsequently developed in 2 intensive-arm and 3 standard-arm participants. No participant underwent kidney transplant for irreversible AKI. The most common reasons for AKI in both intensive and standard groups was dehydration or intravascular volume depletion, followed by hypotension. In both the CKD and non-CKD cohorts, 10.0% of cases of AKI in the intensive arm and 2.3% of cases in the standard arm were thought to be secondary to the intervention. By multivariable analysis, risk factors for time to development of an AKI event included older age, nonwhite race, lower baseline eGFR, and presence of cardiovascular disease at baseline.

The increased frequency of AKI events in the intensive arm may have been caused by the lower baseline systolic BP that resulted in increased risk for BP decreasing to less than the autoregulatory threshold for kidney perfusion when a volume-depleting illness and/or hypotension occurred. Although participants in the intensive arm had increased risk for AKI events, participants in the intensive arm still had reduced risk for the primary SPRINT outcome and all-cause mortality compared with those in the standard arm. These findings help in interpreting the risk-benefit ratio of the SPRINT results and are important to consider when developing clinical guidelines for the management of hypertension.

BIOMARKERS OF KIDNEY INJURY

A nested case-control study within SPRINT compared kidney damage biomarkers between incident CKD participants and matched control participants, as well as participants in the intensive versus standard BP groups at baseline and at 1 year.[25] Higher concentrations of urinary albumin, kidney injury molecule-1, and monocyte chemoattractant protein-1 at baseline were significantly associated with greater odds of incident CKD. After 1 year of BP intervention, participants with incident CKD in the intensive control group had greater decreases in albumin-creatinine ratio, interleukin-18, anti–chitinase-3-like protein 1 (YKL-40), and uromodulin than the matched control participants. Compared with the standard group, those in the intensive group had significantly greater decreases in albumin-creatinine ratio, β-microglobulin, α1-microglobulin, YKL-40, and uromodulin. These findings suggest that incident CKD may reflect benign changes in renal blood flow rather than intrinsic renal injury.

ACTION TO CONTROL CARDIOVASCULAR RISK IN DIABETES BLOOD PRESSURE VERSUS SYSTOLIC BLOOD PRESSURE INTERVENTION TRIAL

An obvious question is whether these results are generalizable to patient populations that were not included in the trial(ie, younger patients, patients with low cardiovascular risk, and those with diabetes). The question is particularly relevant in diabetes, because the ACCORD BP study, which used the same BP targets as SPRINT, did not show a significant difference in the primary cardiovascular outcome between the intensive and standard groups in patients with diabetes. The differences between the 2 trials are detailed in **Table 1**. Compared with SPRINT, ACCORD BP had a complex factorial design, enrolled a lesser number of patients, and excluded patients with creatinine level greater than 1.5 mg/dL. However,

Table 1
Comparison of the action to control cardiovascular risk in diabetes blood pressure trial and systolic blood pressure intervention trial

	ACCORD BP (Intensive vs Standard)	SPRINT (Intensive vs Standard)
Design	RCT, 2 × 2 factorial design	RCT
Number of Participants	4733	9361
Main Inclusion	• Type 2 DM • SBP 130–180 mm Hg • 40 y and older (upper age limit of 79 y)	• SBP 130–180 mm Hg • 50 y and older
Main Exclusion	• Serum creatinine >1.5 mg/dL	• Stroke • DM
Follow-up	Mean follow-up, 4.7 y	Median follow-up, 3.2 y
Age, Mean (y)	62.2	67.9
Female (%)	47.7	35.6
Black (%)	24.1	29.9
Mean eGFR (mL/min/1.73 m^2)	91.6 ± 28.8	71.7 ± 20.6
Mean Achieved Systolic BP (mm Hg)	119.3 vs 133.5	121.5 vs 134.6
Mean Achieved Diastolic BP (mm Hg)	64.4 vs 70.5	68.7 vs 76.3
Mean Number of Medications	3.4 vs 2.1	2.8 vs 1.8
Diuretic of Choice	HCTZ (alone or in combination)	Chlorthalidone
Primary Outcome Definition	Composite of nonfatal MI, nonfatal stroke, and CV mortality	Composite of MI, non-MI ACS, stroke, HF, and CV mortality
Primary Outcomes Results (% event rate/y, HR, 95% CI)	1.87 vs 2.09, 0.88 (0.73–1.06), $P = .20$	1.65 vs 2.19, 0.75 (0.64–0.89), $P<.001$
Adverse Events		
Hypotension, n (%)	17 (0.7) vs 1 (0.04), $P<.001$	158 (3.4) vs 93 (2.0), $P<.001$
Syncope, n (%)	12 (0.5) vs 5 (0.21), $P<.001$	163 (3.5) vs 113 (2.4), $P = .003$
Hypokalemia, n (%)	49 (2.1) vs 27 (1.1), $P = .01$	114 (2.4) vs 74 (1.6), $P = .006$

Abbreviations: ACS, acute coronary syndrome; CV, cardiovascular; HCTZ, hydrochlorothiazide; RCT, randomized controlled trial.

there was a nonsignificant 12% reduction in primary outcome in the intensive group with a wide confidence limit (95% CI, −27% to +6%). Thus, it may be speculated that ACCORD BP was underpowered to detect significant differences in the primary outcome. An analysis after combining data from both trials indicated that effects on individual outcomes were generally consistent in both trials (with no significant heterogeneity noted).[26] Also, the primary composite outcome in ACCORD BP did not include HF, which is particularly sensitive to BP reduction (unlike SPRINT), and ACCORD BP had a higher proportion of events in the primary outcome that are less sensitive to BP reduction. In addition, the factorial design of ACCORD BP involved a simultaneous comparison of intensive versus standard glycemic control,

which may have influenced the effects of BP. A post hoc analysis showed that there was a significant 26% lower risk of primary outcome in ACCORD BP patients in the intensive BP plus standard glycemic control group compared with a standard BP plus standard glycemic control group.[27]

IMPLICATIONS FOR MANAGEMENT

SPRINT is the first large, adequately powered, randomized trial that shows a clear cardiovascular and mortality benefit for intensive BP lowering in patients with cardiovascular risk including CKD, but without a history of DM or stroke, significant proteinuria, or polycystic kidney disease. The cardiovascular benefit in the intensive group was predominantly driven by reduced HF (38% reduction in intensive group, $P = .0002$), and reduced cardiovascular mortality (43% reduction in intensive group, $P = .005$), whereas there was no significant difference between the 2 groups for MI or stroke. The beneficial effect on HF events are consistent with results from other trials, including SHEP or HYVET, all of which showed greatest risk reduction on HF with BP lowering (although to higher levels than SPRINT).

An important aspect of SPRINT is the manner in which BP was measured: an automated BP monitor was used with a protocol of a 5-minute period of rest with average of 3 seated office BP readings. Automated devices have been shown to reduce white-coat effect, and some studies have shown that readings obtained with automated devices correlate better with average daytime blood pressures obtained by ambulatory blood pressure monitoring (ABPM) compared with routine office BP measurements.[28,29] However, in real life, automated devices may not be used and strict protocols for correct BP measurement may not be followed, which could potentially overestimate BP and result in overtreatment. The trial, by design, focused on lowering systolic BP (given the greater prevalence of isolated systolic hypertension with age), and the implications of lowering diastolic BP are unclear. The issue of a J-shaped relationship between diastolic BP and cardiovascular risk is debated in the literature; patients with a diastolic BP of 60 to 65 mm Hg, especially those with existing coronary artery disease, may not tolerate aggressive BP lowering; further analysis of this association (if any) from the SPRINT trial will be helpful.

The risk for adverse events, including hypotension, syncope, electrolyte abnormalities, and AKI, were higher in the intensive group. Some of the adverse events may be related to the effect of antihypertensive medications (such as electrolyte abnormalities, including hyponatremia and hypokalemia caused by diuretic use), and other effects may be related to BP lowering (AKI caused by hypoperfusion and renal ischemia). At this point, the long-term effects of these adverse events, especially on kidney function, are not known. Patients enrolled in clinical trials tend to be healthier than other similar patients; thus, the rate of adverse events reported in the trial may be an underestimate of the adverse event rate that would be seen with routine clinical practice. SPRINT included patients with stage 3 and 4 CKD, but it should be noted that it is a cardiovascular outcomes trial and was not designed to assess CKD progression. It did not include patients with diabetic nephropathy or a high degree of proteinuria.

The risks and benefits of intensive BP control will need to be balanced in individual patients, especially considering the higher incidence of adverse events in the intensive group. It is also unclear whether similar beneficial results would be seen with intensive treatment in a population with low cardiovascular risk; the SPRINT trial design placed emphasis on cardiovascular risk, and the results suggest that risk reduction is proportional to the magnitude of reduction and the absolute baseline cardiovascular risk.

NEW GUIDELINES

The new Guideline for the Prevention, Detection, Evaluation, and Management of High Blood Pressure in Adults issued by the American College of Cardiology and American Heart Association in partnership with 9 other professional associations was published in 2017, addressing a broad range of topics relevant to diagnosis and management of hypertension, and incorporating a wider range of evidence including randomized controlled trials, systematic reviews, and expert opinion.[30] The SPRINT trial results informed many of the recommendations in these guidelines.

Blood Pressure Measurement

Although office-based BP measurement remains the most commonly used modality, it is now increasingly recognized that this snapshot may not be reflective of a patient's true baseline BP. Based on the results of a systematic review commissioned by the guideline committee, out-of-office BP measurements are now recommended for confirmation of the diagnosis of hypertension, and for assessment of response to therapy.

ABPM should be strongly considered as the preferred modality of out-of-office monitoring; home BP monitoring can be done if ABPM is not feasible. ABPM provides additional information on nighttime blood pressure, including the dipping status (defined as normal nighttime BP decrease of 10%–20%). ABPM predicts long-term cardiovascular outcomes independent of office BP, and increased nighttime BP and nondipping have been shown to be independently associated with increased cardiovascular mortality.[31,32] However, despite evidence supporting its use, ABPM is not widely available for a variety of reasons, including expense and minimal reimbursement.

Out-of-office measurements can also detect white-coat hypertension and masked hypertension. White-coat hypertension is defined as BP that is increased in the office but normal in an out-of-office setting, and masked hypertension is defined as BP that is normal in the office and increased in an out-of-office setting. At present, pharmacologic therapy is not recommended to treat white-coat hypertension, and masked hypertension should be managed similarly to sustained hypertension.

In patients with CKD, office BP measurements alone are not ideal to guide hypertension management. Studies have shown a significant prevalence of masked hypertension in this population (apparently normotensive in office and hypertensive out of office)[33,34]; thus, out-of-office measurements should be strongly considered in this population.

The proper technique for BP measurement is appropriately emphasized; correct patient positioning, allowing for a period of rest, and using the appropriate cuff size are all important. However, busy clinical practices may not follow correct technique when measuring BP in the office, with the unintended consequence of misdiagnosis and unnecessary pharmacologic therapy that may result in adverse events. Note that the SPRINT trial, which informed many of the new guideline recommendations, followed a strict protocol of BP measurement with an automated BP device, checking sitting BP 3 times at 1-minute intervals, with the patient alone in the room and without an observer present at many of the sites.[10]

Nonpharmacologic Therapy

Lifestyle modifications should be an integral part of hypertension management in all patients; although not specifically tested in patients with CKD, these interventions would also be appropriate in CKD in the setting of high cardiovascular risk. Lifestyle changes that have been shown to improve BP include dietary modifications (decreased sodium intake, DASH [Dietary Approaches to Stop Hypertension] diet), weight management, physical activity, and moderation in alcohol consumption.[30] In addition, smoking cessation should be emphasized. Note that dietary modifications in patients with CKD, including the DASH diet and use of salt substitutes, should take into account potential risks for hyperkalemia. The DASH diet is high in potassium, calcium, magnesium, and phosphorus, and individual decisions pertaining to diet should be made in patients with CKD, along with additional laboratory surveillance.

Risk-based Approach to Hypertension Management

The algorithm for hypertension management now incorporates objective assessment of cardiovascular risk, specifically estimation of the 10-year atherosclerotic cardiovascular disease (ASCVD) risk, which is defined as risk for coronary heart disease death, nonfatal MI, or fatal or nonfatal stroke.[30] The information required to estimate ASCVD risk includes age, gender, race, total cholesterol, high-density lipoprotein cholesterol, systolic BP, BP-lowering medication use, diabetes status, and smoking status. A 10-year risk of 10% or more is designated as the cutoff between high risk and low risk. Patients with CKD are in the high-risk category.

Blood Pressure Goals

The guidelines recommend a BP goal of less than 130/80 mm Hg for all patients, including the elderly and other disease subgroups, including CKD and diabetes.[30] Although a universal BP goal may simplify decision making, it is important to individualize BP goals, taking into account patient characteristics, lifestyle factors, medication side effects, patient preferences, cost issues, and adherence.

Pharmacologic Therapy

Pharmacologic therapy is recommended in patients with stage 1 hypertension and preexisting cardiovascular disease or 10-year ASCVD risk of 10% or more (patients with CKD are considered high risk), and in those with stage 2 hypertension even if their 10-year ASCVD risk is less than 10%.[30]

First-line pharmacotherapy is based on existing comorbidities. In the absence of compelling indications, the primary pharmacologic agents recommended are thiazide diuretics (preferably chlorthalidone), angiotensin-converting enzyme inhibitors (ACEIs), angiotensin receptor blockers (ARBs), and calcium channel blockers (CCB). In black adults, thiazide diuretics and CCBs are recommended for initial therapy. Treatment with ACEIs or ARBs is recommended in patients with proteinuric CKD, irrespective of race. Starting with a single antihypertensive agent is recommended for stage 1 hypertension with increased cardiovascular risk, and starting with 2 agents (either separately or in fixed-dose combination) is recommended for stage 2 hypertension.

Thiazide-type diuretics include chlorthalidone and indapamide in addition to hydrochlorothiazide (HCTZ). Chlorthalidone is more potent and has a longer duration of action compared with HCTZ, including lowering nighttime BP.[35] Mortality benefits and reduced cardiovascular morbidity has also been reported with the use of chlorthalidone compared with HCTZ.[36,37] One study showed an increased risk of hospitalization for hyponatremia and hypokalemia with the use of chlorthalidone in the elderly.[38] It should be kept in mind that thiazide diuretics are generally ineffective when GFR is less than 30 mL/min/1.73 m^2 and loop diuretics should be used. Short-acting loop diuretics (such as furosemide) should dosed at least twice daily to be effective. Many patients with CKD have resistant hypertension, and diuretics are important in this setting to achieve BP control.

Renin-angiotensin system (RAS) blockers, including ACEIs and ARBs, are effective in reducing proteinuria and slowing progression of CKD by improving glomerular hemodynamics, restoring the altered glomerular barrier function, and limiting the nonhemodynamic effects of angiotensin-II and aldosterone, such as fibrosis and vascular endothelial dysfunction.[39] Studies have shown that these protective effects are, at least in part, independent of the reduction in systemic BP.[40,41] In nondiabetic kidney disease, there is strong evidence from the REIN (Ramipril Efficacy in Nephropathy) and AASK trials that treatment with ACEIs results in slower decline in GFR, and this risk reduction is more pronounced in patients with higher degrees of proteinuria.[42–44] In type 1 diabetes, treatment with the ACEI captopril in patients with overt proteinuria was associated with a 50% decrease in the risk of a combined end point of death, dialysis, or renal transplant. Patients with moderately increased albuminuria and treated with ACEIs also had reduced incidence of progression to overt proteinuria.[45,46] In type 2 diabetes, the IDNT (Irbesartan Diabetic Nephropathy Trial) and RENAAL (Reduction of Endpoints in NIDDM with the Angiotensin II Antagonist Losartan) trials showed that treatment with ARB in patients with overt nephropathy was associated with a significant 20% and 16% decrease in risk, respectively, of the combined end point of death, ESRD, or doubling of serum creatinine level.[47–49] Although there are more data for the use of ARB in type 2 diabetes, the DETAIL (Diabetic Exposed to Telmisartan and Enalapril) study showed that ACEIs were at least as effective as ARBs in providing long-term renal protection in type 2 diabetes and moderately increased albuminuria.[50] Side effects of ACEIs and ARBs include cough (more with ACEIs), angioedema (more with ACEIs), and hyperkalemia. In patients who will benefit from continued RAS inhibition and have had ACEI-related angioedema, ARBs should be used very cautiously.[51] RAS inhibitor therapy can cause a modest increase in creatinine level caused by reduction in intraglomerular pressure. An increase in creatinine level up to 30% that stabilizes in the first 2 months is not necessarily a reason to discontinue therapy. Continued increase in creatinine level should prompt evaluation for excessive decrease in BP (especially with volume depletion caused by concomitant diuretic use) and/or possible bilateral renal artery stenosis. There is no level of GFR or serum creatinine at which an ACEI or ARB is absolutely contraindicated, and this decision should be made on an individual basis in conjunction with a nephrologist. Risks for hyperkalemia should always be kept in mind at lower GFRs. It would be prudent to check serum creatinine and potassium levels within the first week or two after initiation or intensification of renin-angiotensin-aldosterone system (RAAS) inhibition in these patients.

Combination therapy with both ACEIs and ARBs was hypothesized to provide more complete RAAS blockade, with the hope of better cardiovascular and renal outcomes. However, this strategy has been questioned with results from 3 studies, ONTARGET (Ongoing Telmisartan Alone and in Combination With Ramipril Global Endpoint Trial), ALTITUDE (Aliskiren Trial in Type 2 Diabetes Using Cardiorenal Endpoints), and VA NEPHRON-D (Veterans Affairs Nephropathy in Diabetes study), all of which showed worse renal outcomes, hypertension, and hyperkalemia with the use of dual RAAS blockade.[52–55] The combined weight of evidence so far suggests that dual RAAS blockade should not be routinely prescribed. β-Blockers are no longer considered to be optimal initial therapy for hypertension management in the absence of specific indications such as HF or coronary artery disease.[30]

Because more medications will be needed for intensive control, side effects and tolerability of medications with polypharmacy, and potential nonadherence with increasing complexity of medication regimens, should be kept in mind. Lifestyle modifications will need to be emphasized and reinforced, with greater use of combination antihypertensive therapy. Careful monitoring will likely entail more frequent visits and more frequent assessment of renal function and electrolyte levels (participants in the intensive group in the trial were seen every month until the goal was achieved); a team approach using pharmacists and nurse practitioners, along with optimal use of best-practice algorithms and remote monitoring technology, will need to be implemented for efficient and effective care.

REFERENCES

1. Lewington S, Clarke R, Qizilbash N, et al, Prospective Studies Collaboration. Age-specific relevance of usual blood pressure to vascular mortality: a

meta-analysis of individual data for one million adults in 61 prospective studies. Lancet 2002; 360(9349):1903–13.

2. Judd E, Calhoun DA. Management of hypertension in CKD: beyond the guidelines. Adv Chronic Kidney Dis 2015;22(2):116–22.

3. Muntner P, Anderson A, Charleston J, et al, Chronic Renal Insufficiency Cohort (CRIC) Study Investigators. Hypertension awareness, treatment, and control in adults with CKD: results from the chronic renal insufficiency cohort (CRIC) study. Am J Kidney Dis 2010;55(3):441–51.

4. Go AS, Chertow GM, Fan D, et al. Chronic kidney disease and the risks of death, cardiovascular events, and hospitalization. N Engl J Med 2004; 351:1296–305.

5. SHEP Cooperative Research Group. Prevention of stroke by antihypertensive drug treatment in older persons with isolated systolic hypertension: final results of the Systolic Hypertension in the Elderly Program (SHEP). JAMA 1991;265:3255–64.

6. Beckett NS, Peters R, Fletcher AE, et al. Treatment of hypertension in patients 80 years of age or older. N Engl J Med 2008;358:1887–98.

7. JATOS Study Group. Principal results of the Japanese trial to assess optimal systolic blood pressure in elderly hypertensive patients (JATOS). Hypertens Res 2008;31:2115–27.

8. Ogihara T, Saruta T, Rakugi H, et al. Target blood pressure for treatment of isolated systolic hypertension in the elderly: Valsartan in Elderly Isolated Systolic Hypertension study. Hypertension 2010;56: 196–202.

9. Liu L, Zhang Y, Liu G, et al. The Felodipine Event Reduction (FEVER) Study: a randomized longterm placebo-controlled trial in Chinese hypertensive patients. J Hypertens 2005;23:2157–72.

10. Horowitz B, Miskulin D, Zager P. Epidemiology of hypertension in CKD. Adv Chronic Kidney Dis 2015; 22(2):88–95.

11. Appel LJ, Wright JT Jr, Greene T, et al, AASK Collaborative Research Group. Intensive blood-pressure control in hypertensive chronic kidney disease. N Engl J Med 2010;363(10):918–29.

12. Sarnak MJ, Greene T, Wang X, et al. The effect of a lower target blood pressure on the progression of kidney disease: long-term follow-up of the modification of diet in renal disease study. Ann Intern Med 2005;142(5):342–51.

13. Wright JT Jr, Bakris G, Greene T, et al, African American Study of Kidney Disease and Hypertension Study Group. Effect of blood pressure lowering and antihypertensive drug class on progression of hypertensive kidney disease: results from the AASK trial. JAMA 2002;288:2421–31.

14. Upadhyay A, Earley A, Haynes SM, et al. Systematic review: blood pressure target in chronic kidney disease and proteinuria as an effect modifier. Ann Intern Med 2011;154(8):541–8.

15. Kovesdy CP, Lu JL, Molnar MZ, et al. Observational modeling of strict vs conventional blood pressure control in patients with chronic kidney disease. JAMA Intern Med 2014;174(9):1442–9.

16. Cushman WC, Evans GW, Byington RP, et al. Effects of intensive blood-pressure control in type 2 diabetes mellitus. N Engl J Med 2010;362:1575–85.

17. Benavente OR, Coffey CS, Conwit R, et al. Blood-pressure targets in patients with recent lacunar stroke: the SPS3 randomised trial. Lancet 2013; 382:507–15.

18. James PA, Oparil S, Carter BL, et al. 2014 evidence-based guideline for the management of high blood pressure in adults: report from the panel members appointed to the Eighth Joint National Committee (JNC 8). JAMA 2014;311(5):507–20 [Erratum appears in JAMA 2014;311(17):1809].

19. Wheeler DC, Becker GJ. Summary of KDIGO guideline. What do we really know about management of blood pressure in patients with chronic kidney disease? Kidney Int 2013;83(3):377–83.

20. Weber MA, Schiffrin EL, White WB, et al. Clinical practice guidelines for the management of hypertension in the community: a statement by the American Society of hypertension and the International Society of hypertension. J Clin Hypertens (Greenwich) 2014;16(1):14–26.

21. Ambrosius WT, Sink KM, Foy CG, et al. The design and rationale of a multicenter clinical trial comparing two strategies for control of systolic blood pressure: the Systolic Blood Pressure Intervention Trial (SPRINT). Clin Trials 2014;11:532–46.

22. SPRINT Research Group, Wright JT Jr, Williamson JD, Whelton PK, et al. A randomized trial of intensive versus standard blood-pressure control. N Engl J Med 2015;373(22):2103–16.

23. Cheung AK, Rahman M, Reboussin DM, et al, SPRINT Research Group. Effects of intensive BP control in CKD. J Am Soc Nephrol 2017;28(9): 2812–23.

24. Rocco MV, Sink KM, Lovato LC, et al, SPRINT Research Group. Effects of intensive blood pressure treatment on acute kidney injury events in the systolic blood pressure intervention trial (SPRINT). Am J Kidney Dis 2018;71(3):352–61.

25. Zhang WR, Craven TE, Malhotra R, et al, SPRINT Research Group. Kidney damage biomarkers and incident chronic kidney disease during blood pressure reduction: a case-control study. Ann Intern Med 2018;169(9):610–8.

26. Perkovic V, Rodgers A. Redefining blood-pressure targets–SPRINT starts the Marathon. N Engl J Med 2015;373(22):2175–8.

27. Margolis KL, O'Connor PJ, Morgan TM, et al. Outcomes of combined cardiovascular risk factor

management strategies in type 2 diabetes: the ACCORD randomized trial. Diabetes Care 2014; 37(6):1721–8.

28. Myers MG, Godwin M. Automated office blood pressure. Can J Cardiol 2012;28:341–6.

29. Myers MG, Godwin M, Dawes M, et al. Conventional versus automated measurement of blood pressure in primary care patients with systolic hypertension: randomised parallel design controlled trial. BMJ 2011;342:d286.

30. Whelton PK, Carey RM, Aronow WS, et al. 2017 ACC/AHA/AAPA/ABC/ACPM/AGS/APhA/ASH/ASPC/ NMA/PCNA guideline for the prevention, detection, evaluation, and management of high blood pressure in adults: a report of the American College of Cardiology/American Heart Association task force on clinical practice guidelines. Hypertension 2018;71(6): e13–115.

31. Piper MA, Evans CV, Burda BU, et al. Diagnostic and predictive accuracy of blood pressure screening methods with consideration of rescreening intervals: a systematic review for the US Preventive Services Task Force. Ann Intern Med 2015;162(3):192–204.

32. Boggia J, Li Y, Thijs L, et al, International Database on Ambulatory blood pressure monitoring in relation to Cardiovascular Outcomes (IDACO) investigators. Prognostic accuracy of day versus night ambulatory blood pressure: a cohort study. Lancet 2007; 370(9594):1219–29.

33. Pogue V, Rahman M, Lipkowitz M, et al, African American Study of Kidney Disease and Hypertension Collaborative Research Group. Disparate estimates of hypertension control from ambulatory and clinic blood pressure measurements in hypertensive kidney disease. Hypertension 2009; 53(1):20–7.

34. Drawz PE, Alper AB, Anderson AH, et al, Chronic Renal Insufficiency Cohort Study Investigators. Masked hypertension and elevated nighttime blood pressure in CKD: prevalence and association with target organ damage. Clin J Am Soc Nephrol 2016;11(4):642–52.

35. Ernst ME, Carter BL, Goerdt CJ, et al. Comparative antihypertensive effects of hydrochlorothiazide and chlorthalidone on ambulatory and office blood pressure. Hypertension 2006;47(3):352–8.

36. Roush GC, Holford TR, Guddati AK. Chlorthalidone compared with hydrochlorothiazide in reducing cardiovascular events: systematic review and network meta-analyses. Hypertension 2012; 59(6):1110.

37. Dorsch MP, Gillespie BW, Erickson SR, et al. Chlorthalidone reduces cardiovascular events compared with hydrochlorothiazide: a retrospective cohort analysis. Hypertension 2011;57(4):689.

38. Dhalla IA, Gomes T, Yao Z, et al. Chlorthalidone versus hydrochlorothiazide for the treatment of hypertension in older adults: a population-based cohort study. Ann Intern Med 2013;158(6):447.

39. Taal MW, Brenner BM. Renoprotective benefits of RAS inhibition: from ACEI to angiotensin II antagonists. Kidney Int 2000;57:1803–17.

40. Atkins RC, Briganti EM, Lewis JB, et al. Proteinuria reduction and progression to renal failure in patients with type 2 diabetes mellitus and overt nephropathy. Am J Kidney Dis 2005;45:281–7.

41. de Zeeuw D, Remuzzi G, Parving HH, et al. Proteinuria, a target for renoprotection in patients with type 2 diabetic nephropathy: lessons from RENAAL. Kidney Int 2004;65:2309–20.

42. Randomised placebo-controlled trial of effect of ramipril on decline in glomerular filtration rate and risk of terminal renal failure in proteinuric, nondiabetic nephropathy. The GISEN Group (Gruppo Italiano di Studi Epidemiologici in Nefrologia). Lancet 1997;349:1857–63.

43. Ruggenenti P, Perna A, Gherardi G, et al. Renoprotective properties of ACE-inhibition in non-diabetic nephropathies with non-nephrotic proteinuria. Lancet 1999;354:359–64.

44. Agodoa LY, Appel L, Bakris GL, et al, African American Study of Kidney Disease and Hypertension (AASK) Study Group. Effect of ramipril vs amlodipine on renal outcomes in hypertensive nephrosclerosis: a randomized controlled trial. JAMA 2001; 285(21):2719–28.

45. Lewis EJ, Hunsicker LG, Bain RP, et al. The effect of angiotensin-converting enzyme inhibition in diabetic nephropathy. The Collaborative Study Group. N Engl J Med 1993;329:1456–62.

46. Viberti G, Mogensen CE, Groop LC, et al. Effect of captopril on progression to clinical proteinuria in patients with insulin-dependent diabetes mellitus and microalbuminuria. European Microalbuminuria Captopril Study Group. JAMA 1994;271: 275–9.

47. Lewis EJ, Hunsicker LG, Clarke WR, et al, The Collaborative Study Group. Renoprotective effect of the angiotensin-receptor antagonist irbesartan in patients with nephropathy due to type 2 diabetes. N Engl J Med 2001;345(12):851–60.

48. Brenner BM, Copper ME, de Zeeuw D, et al, RENAAL study investigators. Effects of losartan on renal and cardiovascular outcomes in patients with type 2 diabetes and nephropathy. N Engl J Med 2001;345:861–9.

49. Pohl MA, Blumenthal S, Cordonnier DJ, et al. Independent and additive impact of blood pressure control and angiotensin II receptor blockade on renal outcomes in the irbesartan diabetic nephropathy trial: clinical implications and limitations. J Am Soc Nephrol 2005;16(10):3027–37.

50. Barnett AH, Bain SC, Bouter P, et al, Diabetics Exposed to Telmisartan and Enalapril Study Group.

Angiotensin—receptor blockade versus converting-enzyme inhibition in type 2 diabetes and nephropathy. N Engl J Med 2004;351:1952–61.

51. Sharma P, Nagarajan VQ. Can an ARB be given to patients who have had angioedema on an ACE inhibitor? Cleve Clin J Med 2013;80:755–7.

52. ONTARGET Investigators, Yusuf S, Teo KK, Pogue J, et al. Telmisartan, ramipril, or both in patients at high risk for vascular events. N Engl J Med 2008;358:1547–59.

53. Mann JF, Schmieder RE, McQueen M, et al. Renal outcomes with telmisartan, ramipril, or both, in people at high vascular risk (the ONTARGET study): a multicentre, randomised, double-blind, controlled trial. Lancet 2008;372:547–53.

54. Mann JF, Anderson C, Gao P, et al, ONTARGET Investigators. Dual inhibition of the renin-angiotensin system in high-risk diabetes and risk for stroke and other outcomes: results of the ONTARGET trial. J Hypertens 2013;31:414–21.

55. Parving HH, Brenner BM, McMurray JJ, et al, ALTITUDE Investigators. Cardiorenal end points in a trial of aliskiren for type 2 diabetes. N Engl J Med 2012;367:2204–13.

Sudden Cardiac Death in End-Stage Renal Disease

Page V. Salenger, MD

KEYWORDS

- Sudden cardiac death • Dialysis • Arrhythmia monitoring

KEY POINTS

- Sudden cardiac death in patients with end-stage renal disease is common and can be multifactorial event.
- Future studies and directions need to direct efforts in decreasing the risk of sudden cardiac death and improve associated outcomes.
- There remains much work to be done to elucidate the underlying pathophysiology, mechanisms, and treatment of sudden cardiac death in patients with end-stage renal disease.

INTRODUCTION

Sudden cardiac death (SCD) remains a challenging problem in the end-stage renal disease (ESRD) population. Cardiovascular disease accounts for nearly one-half of all deaths in this group of patients, with more than one-quarter of deaths attributed to SCD.[1] The incidence also seems to be higher in the United States as compared with other Western countries, although this finding may be based on differences in reporting methodology or patient populations.[2] One of the issues associated with SCD reporting lies in its definition; SCD has at times been reported as equivalent to "sudden cardiac arrest" (SCA), regardless of whether or not the event is fatal.

In 2006, the American College of Cardiology/American Heart Association/Heart Rhythm Society defined SCA as the "sudden cessation of cardiac activity so that the victim becomes unresponsive, with no normal breathing and no signs of circulation," thus implying successful resuscitation of the patient. The 2006 statement reads "SCD should not be used to describe events that are not fatal."[3] Another reporting flaw is deaths that are unwitnessed are typically classified on the Centers for Medicare and Medicaid Services death notification form 2746 as "cardiac arrest"; therefore, the true incidence as well as type of arrhythmia remains speculative. Other definitions of SCD have specified a time limit to symptom onset (eg, 1 hour)[4] or unwitnessed death without a clear noncardiac etiology in a previously asymptomatic patient within the previous 24 hours.[5]

Overall, it seems that although cardiovascular mortality rates in ESRD are slowly decreasing, SCD rates as a percentage of mortality events have actually increased over time. This observation is particularly evident in the first 90 days after initiation of renal replacement therapy. **Fig. 1** shows the different proportions of causes of mortality in dialysis patients in the United States, as adapted from data from the United States Renal Data System (www.usrds.org). A paucity of data in large, randomized, controlled trials persists regarding identification of risk factors, risk stratification, and treatment of SCD. For example, an area of controversy is the management of congestive heart failure in ESRD and the usefulness of implantable loop recorders (ILRs), implantable cardioverters/defibrillators (ICDs), and left ventricular assist devices (LVADs). This lack of experimental data is beginning to change, because

Disclosure Statement: The author has nothing to disclose.
Home Therapies, DCI, 1633 Church Street, Suite 500, Nashville, TN 37203, USA
E-mail address: Page.salenger@dciinc.org

Cardiol Clin 37 (2019) 319–326
https://doi.org/10.1016/j.ccl.2019.04.010

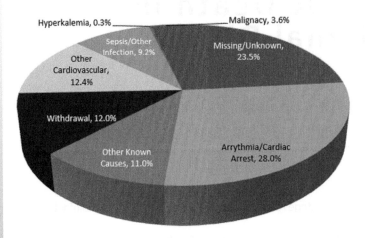

Hyperkalemia, 0.3%

Malignacy, 3.6%

Sepsis/Other Infection, 9.2%

Missing/Unknown, 23.5%

Other Cardiovascular, 12.4%

Withdrawal, 12.0%

Other Known Causes, 11.0%

Arrythmia/Cardiac Arrest, 28.0%

Fig. 1. Causes of death in ESRD. (*Adapted from* the US Renal Data System, 2015 Annual Data Report. Available at https://www.usrds.org/2015/view/Default.aspx.)

recently completed and ongoing trials examine these questions specifically in the dialysis population (see **Fig. 1**).

RISK FACTORS

Generally, risk factors fall into several categories: (1) those specific to ESRD and the uremic state, (2) those specific to the dialysis process itself, and (3) traditional cardiac risk factors. What has become apparent over the last decade is that risk factors in this last category contribute the least to SCD incidence. This finding may explain the disappointing observation that usual therapies preventing SCD in the general population are not efficacious in dialysis patients. As evidenced in the Choices for Healthy Outcomes in Caring for ESRD (CHOICES) study, there is a high prevalence of traditional cardiac risk factors in the ESRD population: these include diabetes mellitus in 54%, low high-density lipoprotein cholesterol levels in 33%, hypertension in 96%, left ventricular hypertrophy (LVH) by electrocardiogram in 22%, and low physical activity in 80%.[6]

Although a low left ventricular ejection fraction (LVEF) in the nondialysis population is considered a risk factor for SCD, the strength of this observation is weakened in ESRD. In 1 study of 80 ESRD deaths secondary to SCD, only 25% had an LVEF of less than or equal to 35%.[7] In fact, it seems that left ventricular mass index may better predict SCD incidence than LVEF. More than 75% of patients starting dialysis have LVH; other factors that may predispose the myocardium to SCD include diffuse myocardial fibrosis (seen by MRI), silent coronary ischemia, and medial vascular calcification with associated arterial stiffening and widened pulse pressure on examination.[8–11] Myocardial fibrosis is thought to predispose to an increased risk of ventricular arrhythmias.

Finally, the dialysis process itself may provide the "trigger" for the generation of dysrhythmias in a vulnerable and diseased myocardium. Over the last decade, multiple studies have consistently shown that intradialytic hypotension (IDH) and/or large interdialytic fluid gains are associated with the development of reversible regional wall motion abnormalities (RWMAs); this phenomenon is also termed myocardial stunning. Efforts to limit volume removal per kilogram of body weight have been implemented in most outpatient clinics; however, in the traditional thrice weekly dialysis model, the nephrologist often must choose between inadequate fluid removal or lengthy treatment times. The problem is compounded in those patients with large fluid gains and/or significant cardiomyopathy.

The presence of RWMAs has been associated not only with higher SCD occurrence, but also with increases in cardiac troponin and N-terminal pro B-type natriuretic peptide. Burton and colleagues,[12] in an observational cohort study of 70 prevalent hemodialysis (HD) patients, found that not only were RWMAs common during dialysis (64%), but they were associated with increased relative mortality and development of low LVEF at 1 year. In a prospective cohort of 230 Chinese peritoneal dialysis (PD) patients followed for 5 years, Wang and colleagues[11] noted that a decreased LVEF and a widened pulse pressure were leading predictors of SCD. They further noted that although cardiac troponin T had a strong association with SCD, no significant relationship was seen between inflammatory markers and SCD, in contrast with other studies.

In addition to RWMAs and IDH, dialysis is associated with oxidative stress, generation of free radical molecules, and increased proinflammatory cytokines. Whether this is additive to already increased levels of reactive oxygen species and reactive carbonyl compounds seen with progressive uremia is unclear.[10] Trials with antioxidant therapy to reduce mortality in ESRD have been disappointing in both the dialysis population and the nondialysis population; for example, treatment of hyperhomocysteinemia with folate.

POTENTIAL INTERVENTIONS

The Secondary Prevention with Antioxidants of Cardiovascular Disease in End Stage Renal Disease (SPACE) study examined the effect of vitamin E supplementation in patients with ESRD with pre-existing cardiovascular disease. Although supplementation was associated with a decreased composite cardiovascular disease incidence, the larger HOPE trial did not duplicate these results.[13] A Cochrane analysis of antioxidants in chronic kidney disease (CKD; including some patients with ESRD), showed possible benefit of cardiovascular disease prevention in ESRD, but without obvious effect on cardiovascular mortality.[14] A study examining acetylcysteine supplementation likewise showed no effect on mortality.[15]

The use of β-hydroxy β-methylglutaryl coenzyme A reductase inhibitors (statins) to treat dyslipidemias illustrates the dilemma of applying traditional treatment methods to patients with ESRD. Despite multiple studies showing the benefit of statins for secondary prevention in the non-ESRD population, the same does not seem to hold true for dialysis patients. There have even been calls to avoid statins entirely in patients with ESRD on the basis of potential acceleration of vascular calcification.[16,17] The Die Deutsche Diabetes Dialyze (4-D) study failed to show a benefit of statins on cardiovascular mortality in diabetic patients with a low-density lipoprotein cholesterol of less than 145 mg/dL; in those with a low-density lipoprotein cholesterol of greater than 145 mg/dL, there seemed to be a benefit in cardiovascular morbidity and mortality, although the study was not originally designed to include these subgroups.[18] In A Study to Evaluate the use of Rosuvastatin (AURORA), again no effect of statins on cardiovascular mortality was proven, although there seemed to be a decrease in cardiovascular events in patients with diabetes receiving rosuvastatin.[19]

The Study of Heart and Renal Protection (SHARP) examined the use of simvastatin and ezetimibe in a combined cohort of patients with CKD who were on dialysis. The 2 drugs together decreased major atherosclerotic events; however, in subgroup analysis, there seemed to be no benefit in the dialysis cohort of more than 3000 patients.[20] Multiple metaanalyses have followed, but failed to show any significant benefit to use of statins in ESRD. As a result, most nephrologists do not initiate statins in their patients; whether or not to discontinue statins in ESRD if the patient has previously been prescribed them is not known. Clear risk factors that would potentially identify those patients with ESRD likely to benefit from statins are lacking. It is felt that this "statin resistance" may be secondary to increased inflammatory stress, which can alter β-hydroxy β-methylglutaryl coenzyme A reductase activity and lead to intracellular lipid accumulation.[21]

ROLE OF ARTIFICIAL HEMODYNAMIC SUPPORT

Similarly, the optimal role of LVADs in preventing SCD in ESRD has not been determined. Initial studies of Medicare claims data of patients with ESRD receiving LVADs suggested extremely high mortality, with average survival after implantation of 16 days.[22,23] However, as technology has advanced, survival in both patients with and without ESRD has improved, although the mortality rates in the former group remain suboptimal.[24] In particular, the shift from early pulsatile flow devices to continuous flow LVADs has resulted in improved survival with fewer complications.[25] Nonetheless, guidelines still recommend against the placement of destination LVADs in patients with ESRD. The use of anticoagulant and antiplatelet therapies can contribute to coagulopathy already present in dialysis patients. Because LVADs produce significant shear stress with subsequent hemolysis, anemia and hyperkalemia can be exaggerated. Acquired von Willebrand disease with associated arteriovenous malformations can be seen with LVADs and increases the risks of gastrointestinal bleeding.[26]

An additional consideration in patients with ESRD is the choice of modality of dialysis in a patient with an LVAD. There are no randomized, controlled trials addressing this question. Theoretically, PD seems more advantageous than HD, given its more continuous nature and decreased hemodynamic instability. There also seems to be a decreased incidence of bacteremia when compared with HD patients with tunneled venous catheters. Placement of the driveline pathway and exit site should avoid the peritoneum, to reduce the risks of peritonitis or cross-contamination with the PD catheter. Because of variability of blood pressure during HD treatments, there is concern of LVAD malfunction and thrombosis, given that newer LVADs are volume dependent.[27]

Successful arteriovenous fistula placement and use has been described in patients with ESRD with LVADs. Future research is still needed to determine if PD is the more appropriate initial dialysis modality, especially because PD is known to preserve residual renal function for a longer period of time than HD.[28]

RESIDUAL RENAL FUNCTION AND ELECTROLYTES

Increasingly, the importance of residual renal function and its influence on survival has become clearer. A reanalysis of data from the Canada-USA Peritoneal Dialysis Study Group (CANUSA) study showed that for each 5 L/wk/1.73 m^2 increase in the residual renal glomerular filtration rate, there was a 12% decrease in the relative risk of death; each 250 mL of urine output was associated with a 36% decrease in overall mortality.[29] The same effect has been noted in HD patients, and newer data suggest that the rate of loss of the glomerular filtration rate may be the more important variable.[30,31] The exact underlying mechanisms are incompletely elucidated, but are thought to be related to volume control (hence reduced LVH), improved small solute and middle molecule clearance, and better controlled anemia and mineral bone disease. Residual renal function is also associated with a decreased inflammatory state and reduced oxidative stress.

An area of relatively recent research is the role of magnesium in reducing SCD risk. Magnesium, which has a well-known role in torsade de pointes, may also attenuate atherosclerotic heart disease and decrease SCD risk. Putative mechanisms include vasodilatation via increased nitric oxide production, decreased platelet aggregation via increased prostaglandin production, and smooth muscle relaxation mediated by calcium channels.[32] This last effect may involve a magnesium-induced decrease in arterial medial calcification. Whether or not this will translate into improved survival in patients with ESRD will require a larger, randomized trial. An observational analysis of 365 European patients with ESRD showed that, for every increase in baseline magnesium of 0.1 mmol/L, there was an associated hazard ratio of 0.85 for all-cause mortality, 0.73 for cardiovascular mortality, and 0.76 for SCD incidence. This association persisted after adjustment for confounding factors.[33] In an observational study of more than 20,000 HD patients, a nearly linear association was noted between serum magnesium levels and decreased mortality, although the relationship with SCD was not significant in adjusted models.[34] The use of oral magnesium supplements or

increased magnesium concentration in the dialysate await larger, randomized trials to confirm this effect.

Another mineral felt to influence SCD incidence in ESRD is calcium. Low dialysate calcium concentrations have a known association with both IDH and QT prolongation. Pun and colleagues,[35,36] in a study of approximately 2000 patients with ESRD (in 1:3 case:control ratio), showed an association between serum calcium, lower dialysate calcium concentration, and the calcium gradient between blood and dialysate. The gradient directly correlated with the risk of cardiac arrest. Further studies may establish that this gradient is more predictive of SCA than the serum calcium level alone.

There was no relationship between drugs that prolong the QT interval and the incidence of SCA.[35,36] Hypercalcemia remains a concern as well, because it may promote vascular calcification. Given these competing risks, the existing weight of opinion in recent guidelines recommends avoidance of calcium based phosphate binders and use of a 2.5 mEq/L calcium concentration in the dialysate. Might reduction in calcium load result in decreased vascular calcification and subsequent reduction in cardiovascular death?

The Evaluation of Cinacalcet Therapy to Lower Cardiovascular Events Trial (EVOLVE) was a randomized, double-blind, placebo-controlled study of nearly 4000 patients with ESRD in multiple countries with secondary hyperparathyroidism, designed to study this question. Patients received the calcimimetic cinacalcet, although statistical power was diminished by high withdrawal rates because of side effects of cinacalcet. SCD accounted for 25% of all deaths. The results were mixed in that cinacalcet somewhat decreased rates of SCD and congestive heart failure after adjustment for baseline characteristics; any decrease in atherosclerotic events was not statistically significant.[37]

The most frequent type of arrhythmia in patients with ESRD with SCA remains a subject of debate. More recent studies shed light on this question. A study in Washington state of 110 cardiac arrests in outpatient dialysis clinics over 14 years showed that SCA was more likely after the longest interdialytic interval, consistent with prior published data. In this study, the majority of SCA occurred during dialysis, with nearly two-thirds of patients sustaining ventricular arrhythmias (primarily fibrillation), an unusually high incidence.[38] Newer data suggest that dialysis vintage may play a role in the type of arrhythmia, with ventricular arrhythmias predominating in newer dialysis patients, and bradycardia and asystole seen more frequently in patients on dialysis for several years. Wong and colleagues[39] followed 50 patients with ESRD with an LVEF of greater than 35% after insertion of an implantable cardiac monitor. After a mean follow-up of 18 months, 16% of patients suffered SCD, all secondary to bradycardia with asystole in 1 patient. Again, these events all occurred during the longest interdialytic interval.

MONITORING DEVICES

The Cardiorenal Arrhythmia Study in Hemodialysis Patients Using Implantable Loop Recorders (CRASH- LR) was a prospective single center study of 30 unselected patients with ESRD with a median dialysis vintage of 45 months.[40] At baseline, only 1 patient had an LVEF of less than 35% and approximately one-fourth of patients had been prescribed beta-blockers. There were 8 deaths, 2 from SCD; 3 patients required pacemaker implantation. Patients reaching the primary endpoint (SCD or pacer) were older, with a lower LVEF and more LVH. Overall, bradyarrhythmias were the dominant, clinically significant rhythm. The authors raise the question of whether or not pacer/ICD placement is truly beneficial in these patients for primary prevention of SCD.

The Monitoring in Dialysis (MiD) study was a multicenter, observational–interventional, prospective cohort study in which patients with ESRD consented to ILR placement. The purpose was to examine frequency and type of "clinically significant arrhythmias" (CSAs) occurring over a 6-month period. CSAs were defined in association with syncope, cardiac arrest or evidence of poor perfusion, and included:

- VT greater than or equal to 115 BPM lasting greater than or equal to 30 seconds
- Bradycardia defined as a heart rate of less than or equal to 40 BPM for greater than or equal to 6 seconds
- Asystole for greater than or equal to 3 seconds
- Symptoms noted by patient correlating with CSAs

The study enrollment was stopped after 66 patients had ILRs implanted. One-third of the patients were from India; there was a greater proportion of diabetic kidney disease and arteriovenous fistula use in these patients.[41] Recently published results were surprising: 67% of patients had CSAs, with 20% bradycardic events and 9% asystole; only 1 incident of ventricular tachycardia occurred as a CSA. CSAs were more frequent during the long interdialytic interval, as well as during the first dialysis session of the week. In this study,

potassium and magnesium flux during treatment did not seem to contribute to incidence of CSAs; however, CSAs were more frequent with calcium dialysate concentration of 2.5 mEq/L, warmer dialysate, and sodium flux.[42] Surprisingly, higher dialysate calcium concentration (>2.5 mEq/L) were associated with fewer CSAs.

More recent studies have implicated bradycardic events and asystole as the predominant rhythm before SCA, as opposed to ventricular dysrhythmias. Upwards of 80% of large cardiovascular trials have excluded patients with ESRD, although this is slowly changing.[43] The availability of leadless implantable cardiac monitors, able to continuously monitor rhythm for several years, will provide improved characterization of the "pre-SCD" state in ESRD. The challenge is to identify those patients at highest risk, because financial limitations will prevent placement of implantable cardiac monitors in all patients. With regard to ICD placement, patients with ESRD have been excluded from major trials, and it is difficult to extrapolate results to patients with ESRD. Herzog and colleagues[44] published a retrospective cohort study in which ICD implantation for secondary prevention was independently associated with a 42% decrease in death risk. Multiple metaanalyses generally show a survival benefit to ICD placement in CKD and ESRD, although not all trials clearly stated if placement was for primary or secondary prevention. It seems that the benefits of ICD placement may decline as one approaches ESRD. Whether or not the placement of ICDs is indicated for the primary prevention of SCD in ESRD is not clear, given competing comorbidities and higher rates of procedural complications.[45–48]

DIALYSIS PROCEDURE AND OTHER TREATMENTS

Cooling of dialysate has long been used by nephrologists to attenuate IDH. There is some evidence that dialysate temperatures of 35°C to 36°C (vs 37°C) may result in the long-term reduction of left ventricular mass index and left ventricular end-diastolic volume.[49] Additionally, small studies of patients with ESRD prone to IDH demonstrate a decrease in RWMAs with cooled dialysate. It remains unanswered if this inexpensive intervention will result in improved clinical outcomes.[50]

One modifiable risk factor that may contribute to SCD risk is dialysate potassium concentration. In the 2012 Dialysis Outcomes and Practice Patterns Study (DOPPS), a significant variation in SCD incidence and dialysate potassium was noted between participating countries. In addition, a higher

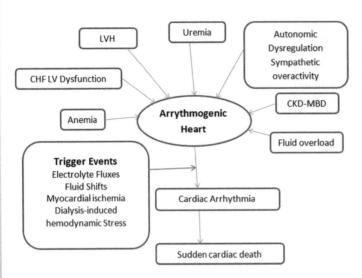

Fig. 2. Potential predisposing factors of SCD. CHF, congestive heart failure; CKD-MBD, chronic kidney disease mineral and bone disorder. (*From* Turakhia, Mintu P, et al. Chronic kidney disease and arrhythmias: conclusions from a Kidney Disease: Improving Global Outcomes (KDIGO) controversies conference. European Heart Journal 2018;39(24):2314–2325; with permission.)

risk of SCD was noted with dialysate potassium concentrations of even less than 3 mEq/mL, with lower predialysis serum potassium a possible additional risk.[2]

In contrast, more recent DOPPS data from more than 55,000 HD patients showed no difference in mortality between dialysate potassium concentrations of 2 and 3 mEq/L.[51] There was, however, an association between hyperkalemia with overall mortality and SCD. In addition to the absolute concentration of potassium in the dialysate, potassium flux itself between the blood and dialysate may heighten the risk of fatal arrhythmias. Logistically, it would be difficult to implement a "potassium profile" for each patient. Unclear as well is whether or not more frequent HD, or PD, both of which would cause smaller variations in potassium levels, are associated with a lower risk of SCD.

The Randomized Aldactone Evaluation Study (RALES) first showed the role of spironolactone use associated with a reduction in cardiovascular events.[52] However, RALES excluded patients with a serum creatinine of more than 2.5 mg/dL. The Dialysis Outcomes Heart Failure Aldactone Study (DOHAS) was a prospective, randomized, controlled, open-label trial in Japan of more than 300 HD patients examining the same question. Low-dose (25 mg/d) spironolactone resulted in a lowering of the incidence of primary outcome (composite of death or hospitalization from cardiovascular or cerebrovascular events) and the secondary outcome (all-cause mortality).[53] Blockade of mineralocorticoid receptors in the myocardium, which are thought to be more highly expressed in renal failure, may constitute the primary mechanistic pathway to SCD occurrence. The recently published results of the Spironolactone in Dialysis (Spin-D) trial demonstrated safe use of spironolactone dosed at 25 mg daily in ESRD, but did not show any improvement in cardiovascular status.[54] These small studies await larger trials of longer duration to better assess ability to improve cardiovascular outcomes. SGLT2 inhibitors have been shown to reduce cardiovascular risk in patients with CKD and diabetes in the Empaglifozin Cardiovascular Outcomes Trial in Type 2 Diabetes and the Canaglifozin Cardiovascular Awareness Program. Ongoing trials will further address this potential benefit, although trials to date have not included patients with ESRD.[55]

SUMMARY

SCD in patients with ESRD is common and can be a multifactorial event. **Fig. 2** outlines a schematic of this complex yet significant problem. Future studies and directions need to direct efforts in reducing the risk of SCD and improve associated outcomes. There remains much work to be done to elucidate the underlying pathophysiology, mechanisms, and treatment of SCD in ESRD[56] (see **Fig. 2**).

REFERENCES

1. Saran R, Li Y, Robinson B, et al. US renal data system 2014 annual data report: epidemiology of kidney disease in the United States. Am J Kidney Dis 2015;66(1 Suppl 1):Svii.
2. Jadool M, Thumma J, Fuller DS, et al. Modifiable practices associated with sudden death among hemodialysis patients in the Dialysis Outcomes and Practice Patterns Study. Clin J Am Soc Nephrol 2012;7(5):765–74.

3. American College of Cardiology/American Heart Association Task Force on Clinical Data Standards (ACC/AHA/HRS writing committee to develop data standards on electrophysiology), Buxton AE, Calkins H, Callans DJ, et al. ACC/AHA/HRS 2006 key data elements and definitions for electrophysiological studies and procedures: a report of the American College of Cardiology/American Heart Association Task Force on Clinical Data Standards (ACC/AHA/HRS writing committee to develop data standards on electrophysiology). Circulation 2006; 114:2534.

4. Mann D, Zipes D, Libby P, et al. Braunwald's Heart Disease: a textbook of cardiovascular medicine. 10th edition. Philadelphia: Elsevier/Saunders; 2015.

5. Herzog CA, Asinger RW, Berger AK, et al. Cardiovascular disease in chronic kidney disease. A clinical update from Kidney Disease: Improving Global Outcomes (KDIGO). Kidney Int 2011;80(6):572–86.

6. Longenecker JC, Coresh J, Powe NR, et al. Traditional cardiovascular disease risk factors in dialysis patients compared with the general population: the CHOICE study. J Am Soc Nephrol 2002;13:1918–27.

7. Bleyer AJ, Hartman J, Brannon PC, et al. Characteristics of sudden death in hemodialysis patients. Kidney Int 2006;69(12):2268–73.

8. Makar MS, Pun PH. Sudden cardiac death among hemodialysis patients. Am J Kidney Dis 2017; 69(5):684–95.

9. Shafi T, Guallar E. Mapping progress in reducing cardiovascular risk with kidney disease. Clin J Am Soc Nephrol 2018;13:1429–31.

10. Hörl WH, Cohen JJ, Harrington JT, et al. Atherosclerosis and uremic retention solutes. Kidney Int 2004; 66:1719.

11. Wang AY, Lam CW, Chan IH, et al. Sudden cardiac death in end stage renal disease patients: a 5 year prospective analysis. Hypertension 2010;56:210–6.

12. Burton JO, Jefferies HJ, Selby NM, et al. Hemodialysis induced cardiac injury: determinants and associated outcomes. Clin J Am Soc Nephrol 2009;4: 914–20.

13. Boaz M, Smetana S, Weinstein T, et al. Secondary prevention with antioxidants of cardiovascular disease in end stage renal disease (SPACE): randomized placebo controlled trial. Lancet 2000;356: 1213–8.

14. Jun M, Venkataraman V, Razavian M, et al. Antioxidants for chronic kidney disease. Cochrane Database Syst Rev 2012;(10):CD008176.

15. Tepel M, van der Giet M, Statz M, et al. The antioxidant acetylcysteine reduces cardiovascular events in patients with end-stage renal failure: a randomized, controlled trial. Circulation 2003;107(7): 992–5.

16. De Vriese AS. Should statins be banned from dialysis? J Am Soc Nephrol 2017;10:1681.

17. Chen Z, Qureshi AR, Parini P, et al. Does statins promote vascular calcification in chronic kidney disease? Eur J Clin Invest 2017;47(2):137–48.

18. März W, Genser B, Drechsler C, et al, German Diabetes and Dialysis Study Investigators. Atorvastatin and low density lipoprotein cholesterol in type 2 diabetes mellitus patients on hemodialysis. Clin J Am Soc Nephrol 2011;6(6):1316–25.

19. Fellstrom BC, Jardine AG, Schmieder RE, et al. Rosuvastatin and cardiovascular events in patients undergoing hemodialysis. N Engl J Med 2009;360: 1395–407.

20. Baigent C, Landray MJ, Reith C, et al, SHARP Investigators. The effects of lowering LDL cholesterol with simvastatin plus ezetimibe in patients with chronic kidney disease (Study of Heart and Renal Protection): a randomized placebo-controlled trial. Lancet 2011;377(9784):2181–92.

21. Chen Y, Zhao L, Li Q, et al. Inflammatory stress reduces the effectiveness of statins in the kidney by disrupting HMGCoA reductase feedback regulation. Nephrol Dial Transplant 2014;29(10):1864–78.

22. Bansal N, Hailpern SM, Katz R, et al. Outcomes associated with left ventricular assist devices among recipients with and without end stage renal disease. JAMA Intern Med 2018;178(2):204–9.

23. Allar D. End stage kidney patients who receive LVADs likely to die before discharge. Cardiovascular Business 2017.

24. Walther CP, Winkelmayer WC, Deswal A, et al. Trends in left ventricular assist device implantation and associated mortality among patients with and without ESRD. Am J Kidney Dis 2018;72(4):620–2.

25. Roehm B, Vest AR, Weiner DE, et al. Left ventricular assist devices, kidney disease and dialysis. Am J Kidney Dis 2018;71(2):257–66.

26. Ross DW, Stevens GR, Wanchoo R, et al. Left ventricular assist devices and the kidney. Clin J Am Soc Nephrol 2018;13(2):348–55.

27. Tromp TR, de Jonge N, Joles JA. Left ventricular assist devices: a kidney's perspective. Heart Fail Rev 2015;20(4):519–32.

28. Thomas BA, Logar CM, Anderson AE, et al. Renal replacement therapy in congestive heart failure requiring left ventricular assist device augmentation. Perit Dial Int 2012;32(4):386–92.

29. Bargman JM, Thorpe KE, Churchill DN, CANUSA Peritoneal Dialysis Study Group. Relative contribution of residual renal function and peritoneal clearance to adequacy of dialysis: reanalysis of CANUSA. J Am Soc Nephrol 2001;12(10):2158–62.

30. Shemin D, Bostom AG, Laliberty P, et al. Residual kidney function and mortality risk in hemodialysis patients. Am J Kidney Dis 2001;38(1):85–90.

31. Liao CT, Chen YM, Shiao CC, et al. Rate of decline of residual renal function is associated with all-cause mortality and technique failure in patients on

long-term peritoneal dialysis. Nephrol Dial Transplant 2009;24:2909–14.

32. Geiger H, Wanner C. Magnesium in disease. Clin Kidney J 2012;5(Suppl 1):i25–38.

33. De Roij van Zuijdewljn CL, Grooteman MP, Bots ML, et al. Serum magnesium and sudden death in European hemodialysis patients. PLoS One 2015;10(11): e0143104.

34. Lacson E Jr, Wang W, Ma L, et al. Serum magnesium and mortality in hemodialysis patients in the United States: a cohort study. Am J Kidney Dis 2015; 66(6):1055–66.

35. Pun PH, Lehrich RW, Honeycutt EF, et al. Modifiable risk factors associated with sudden cardiac arrest within hemodialysis clinics. Kidney Int 2011;79: 218–27.

36. Pun PH, Horton JR, Middleton JP, et al. Dialysate calcium concentrations and the risk of sudden cardiac arrest in hemodialysis patients. Clin J Am Soc Nephrol 2013;8(5):797–803.

37. Wheeler DC, London GM, Parfrey PS, et al. Effects of cinacalcet on atherosclerotic and non-atherosclerotic cardiovascular events in patients receiving hemodialysis: the evaluation of cinacalcet HCL therapy to lower cardiovascular events (EVOLVE) trial. J Am Heart Assoc 2014;3(6): e001363.

38. Davis TR, Young BA, Eisenberg MS, et al. Outcome of cardiac arrests attended by emergency medical services staff at community outpatient dialysis centers. Kidney Int 2008;73(8):933–9.

39. Wong MCG, Kalman JM, Pedagogos E, et al. Temporal distribution of arrhythmic events in chronic kidney disease: highest incidence in the long interdialytic period. Heart Rhythm 2015;12(10): 2047–55.

40. Roberts PR, Zachariah D, Morgan JM, et al. Monitoring of arrhythmia and sudden death in a hemodialysis population: the CRASH-ILR Study. PLoS One 2017;12(12):e0188713.

41. Charytan DM, Foley R, McCullough PA, et al. Arrhythmias and sudden death in hemodialysis patients: protocol and baseline characteristics of the monitoring in dialysis study. Clin J Am Soc Nephrol 2016;11:721–34.

42. Roy-Chaudhury P, Tumlin JA, Koplan BA, et al. Primary outcomes of the Monitoring in Dialysis Study indicate that clinically significant arrhythmias are common in hemodialysis patients and related to dialytic cycle. Kidney Int 2018;93(4):941–51.

43. Charytan D, Kuntz RE. The exclusion of patients with chronic kidney disease from clinical trials in coronary artery disease. Kidney Int 2006;70(11): 2021–30.

44. Herzog CA, Li S, Weinhandl ED, et al. Survival of dialysis patients after cardiac arrest and the impact of implantable cardioverter-defibrillators. Kidney Int 2005;68(2):812–25.

45. Sakhiya R, Keebler M, Lai TS, et al. Meta-analysis of mortality in dialysis patients with an implantable cardioverter defibrillator. Am J Cardiol 2009;103(5): 735–41.

46. Boriani G, Savelieva I, Dan GA, et al. Chronic kidney disease in patients with cardiac rhythm disturbances or implantable electrical devices: clinical significance and implications for decision making-a position paper of the European Heart Rhythm Association endorsed by the Heart Rhythm Society and the Asia Pacific Heart Rhythm Society. Europace 2015;17:1169–96.

47. Chen T-H, Wo HT, Chang PC, et al. A meta-analysis of mortality in end-stage renal disease patients receiving implantable cardioverter defibrillators (ICDs). PLoS One 2014;9(7):e99418.

48. Makki N, Swaminathan PD, Hanmer J, et al. Do implantable cardioverter defibrillators improve survival in patients with chronic kidney disease at high risk of sudden cardiac death? A meta-analysis of observational studies. Europace 2014; 16:55–62.

49. Toth-Manikowski SM, Sozio SM. Cooling dialysate during in-center hemodialysis: beneficial and deleterious effects. World J Nephrol 2016;5(2):166–71.

50. Selby NM, Burton JO, Chesterton LJ, et al. Dialysis-induced regional left ventricular dysfunction is ameliorated by cooling the dialysate. Clin J Am Soc Nephrol 2006;1(6):1216–25.

51. Karaboyas A, Zee J, Brunelli SM, et al. Dialysate potassium, serum potassium, mortality, and arrhythmia events in hemodialysis: results from the dialysis outcomes and practice patterns study (DOPPS). Am J Kidney Dis 2017;69(2):266–77.

52. Pitt B, Zannad F, Remme WJ, et al. The effect of spironolactone on morbidity and mortality in patients with severe heart failure. N Engl J Med 1999;341: 709–17.

53. Matsumoto Y, Mori Y, Kageyama S, et al. Spironolactone reduces cardiovascular and cerebrovascular morbidity and mortality in hemodialysis patients. J Am Coll Cardiol 2014;63(6):528–36.

54. Charytan DM, Himmelfarb J, Ikizler TA, et al. Safety and cardiovascular efficacy of spironolactone in dialysis-dependent ESRD (SPin-D): a randomized, placebo-controlled, multiple dosage trial. Kidney Int 2018;95(4):973–82.

55. Pecoits-Filho R, Perkovic V. Are SGLT2 inhibitors ready for prime time for CKD? Clin J Am Soc Nephrol 2018;13(2):318–20.

56. Turakhia MP, Blankestijn PJ, Carrero JJ, et al. Chronic kidney disease and arrhythmias: conclusions from a kidney disease: improving global outcomes (KDIGO) controversies conference. Eur Heart J 2018;39(24):2314–25.

Apolipoprotein L1, Cardiovascular Disease and Hypertension
More Questions than Answers

Niralee Patel, MD, Girish N. Nadkarni, MD, MPH*

KEYWORDS

• Cardiovascular disease • Hypertension • Kidney disease

KEY POINTS

• *APOL1* risk variants are common in persons of African ancestry (including African Americans and Hispanic Americans) and are one of the most powerful disease variants identified to date in terms of frequency and effect size for kidney disease.
• The association of *APOL1* with other linked diseases, such as cardiovascular disease and hypertension, is still controversial.
• These studies are essential to understanding the role that testing will play in clinical outcomes, and ultimately what the benefit to patients is, the ultimate goal of translational research.

APOLIPOPROTEIN L1 AND PARASITES: AN EXAMPLE OF EVOLUTIONARY ADAPTATION

The Apolipoprotein L1 (*APOL1*) gene, located on the short arm of chromosome 22, is only found in humans and closely related primate species.[1] As part of the innate immunity mechanism, *APOL1* protects humans against African sleeping sickness, which is a protozoan parasitic infection caused by *Trypanosoma brucei*. This parasite is transmitted by the tsetse fly, and the disease has a prevalence of 11% in sub-Saharan Africa. *APOL1* on high-density lipoprotein particles is taken up by the trypanosome cells,[2] causes osmotic swelling of the lysosome by means of chloride influx, and then, ultimately, lysis of the parasite.

There are 3 components to *APOL1* causing trypanolytic activity, a pore-forming domain, a pH-sensitive membrane-addressing domain, and the serum resistance-associated protein (SRA)-interacting domain. However, 2 species, *Trypanosoma brucei rhodesiense* in East Africa and *Trypanosoma brucei gambiense* in West Africa, have separately evolved resistance to the trypanolytic activity of *APOL1* through the generation of a virulence factor called SRA, which can inactivate *APOL1* protein and prevent its trypanolytic activity.[3] As a means of evolutionary survival adaptation, variants arose in *APOL1* (G1/G2 variants) that encode forms of *APOL1* that evade SRA. This likely confers a selective advantage to African American individuals carrying these variants, causing a selection advantage.

POPULATION GENETICS AND WORLDWIDE DISTRIBUTION OF *APOL1*

Chromosome 22 has been a genetic region of interest well before the *APOL1* risk variants were discovered. Initially, variants of the myosin heavy chain 9 (MYH9), also on chromosome 22, which

Disclosure statement: Dr G.N. Nadkarni is supported by a career development award from the National Institutes of Health (NIH) (K23DK107908) and is also supported by R01DK108803, U01HG007278, U01HG009610, and 1U01DK116100. The remaining authors have nothing to disclose.
Division of Nephrology, Icahn School of Medicine at Mount Sinai, 1 Gustave L. Levy Pl, New York, NY 10029, USA
* Corresponding author. One Gustave Levy Place, Box 1243, New York, NY 10029.
E-mail address: girish.nadkarni@mountsinai.org

were in close proximity to *APOL1*, were considered to be associated with the increased risk of nondiabetic end-stage renal disease (ESRD) and focal segmental glomerulosclerosis (FSGS) in African American individuals.[4] However, a novel form of genetic analysis, called admixture mapping, led to the discovery that the increased risk of FSGS initially attributed to *MYH9* were likely due to 2 sequence variants (G1 and G2) in the adjacent *APOL1* gene.[5] G1 risk variant has 2 missense mutations (rs73885319 and rs60910145) in high linkage disequilibrium, whereas G2 has 6 base pair deletions (rs71785313), both resulting in protein alteration[6] (**Fig. 1**).

The G1 and G2 risk variants seem to be the most common in western sub-Saharan Africa, as observed in the Human Genome Diversity Project and International HapMap Project. These variants both have highest frequencies Ghana and Nigeria (>40% for G1 and 6%–24% for G2). G1 variants are found in 20% of African individuals, whereas G2 variants are found in 15%. Approximately 14% to 16% of individuals from Africa carry both *APOL1* variants (G1/G1, G2/G2, or G1/G2), known to be the high-risk genotypes.

However, the frequency of these variants differs by countries within the African continent. A study by Behar and colleagues[7] showed that the prevalence of *APOL1* variants is much lower than in West Africa. Similarly, a study focusing on South Africans with mixed ancestry found that risk alleles were carried in ~16%, with a frequency of only 1% for 2 risk alleles, which is lower than the prevalence in African Americans.[8] This variability of prevalence of *APOL1* risk variants in Africa is likely because of the low prevalence of the tsetse fly in regions outside West Africa.

On the other hand, individuals who are not from the African continent, and those who do not self-identify as African American, may have high frequencies of *APOL1* risk variants owing to worldwide patterns of migration and the sharing of recent African ancestry. This may be especially true of Hispanic Americans and individuals from Caribbean countries who share recent African ancestry. A recent paper, using linked genetic and demographic data from the Population Architecture using Genetics and Epidemiology-II consortium, showed that other populations had increased frequencies of the *APOL1* risk genotype, including Jamaican, Barbadian, Grenadian, and Brazilian from Salvador (>10% to 22%); Trinidadian, Panamanian, Honduran, Haitian, Garifunan, and Palenque (>5% to 10%); and Guyanese, Dominican, Peruvian, Belizean, and Native American (1%–5%).[9] A recent tool to estimate frequency of APOL1 risk genotype has been developed at http://APOL1.org. Thus,

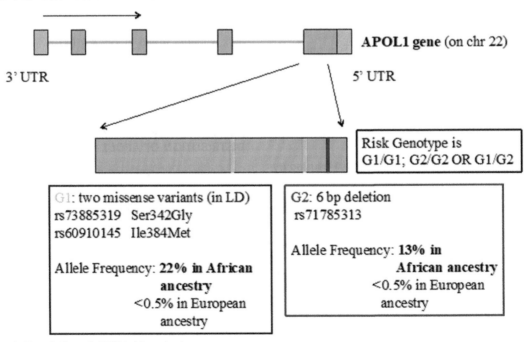

Kidney Disease Burden in African Ancestry Hypertensive Patients: *APOL1* Risk Variants G1 and G2

Fig. 1. Description of *APOL1* risk variants.

APOL1 risk variants exist at appreciable frequencies among many populations of persons in the Americas who share Western African genetic ancestry, but who may not self-identify as African or African American. Previous studies have also shown that the APOL1 risk genotype is also linked to kidney disease outcomes in Hispanic Americans who do not identify themselves as African American[10] (see **Fig. 1**).

APOL1 AND THE SPECTRUM OF KIDNEY DISEASE

It has been shown, by several epidemiologic studies, that African Americans have a 2-fold higher risk of ESRD compared with European Americans, even when accounting for environmental, socioeconomic, and comorbid risk factors.[11–13]

Since the seminal paper showing the association of APOL1 risk variants with FSGS,[5] a plethora of literature has shown its consistent association with kidney disease phenotypes. The association with FSGS was confirmed by Kopp and colleagues,[14] who found that those with *APOL1* high-risk genotype had a younger age of onset of disease by almost 6 years. In addition, they showed that individuals with *APOL1* high-risk genotype had 29-fold odds of developing human immunodeficiency virus-associated nephropathy (HIVAN). This suggests that HIVAN in African ancestry individuals is unlikely to develop in the absence of APOL1 high-risk genotype. This is further supported by the fact that individuals with Ethiopian ancestry and HIV have a low prevalence of HIVAN, and that they have an absence of *APOL1* risk variants.[7]

There have been several studies linking *APOL1* high-risk genotype with various kidney phenotypes, including chronic kidney disease (CKD),[15] earlier age of dialysis initiation,[16,17] and proteinuria. A seminal study by Parsa and colleagues[18] in 2 separate cohorts (the African American Study of Kidney Disease and Hypertension [AASK] and Chronic Renal Insufficiency) showed that *APOL1* high-risk genotype was strongly associated with CKD progression, regardless of baseline proteinuria or history of type 2 diabetes. A summary of kidney phenotypes and histopathology findings associated with APOL1 is shown in **Fig. 2**.

This epidemiologic evidence is further bolstered by several elegant mechanistic studies on how *APOL1* causes kidney injury. The putative mechanisms include activation of stress kinases and AMP-activated protein kinase,[20] endolysosomal trafficking/autophagic flux,[21] mitochondrial dysfunction,[22] and outside-in cellular signaling.[23]

APOL1 AND CARDIOVASCULAR DISEASE: THE PLOT THICKENS

As opposed to the clear links between *APOL1* and kidney disease, the relationship with cardiovascular disease (CVD) is much more convoluted and

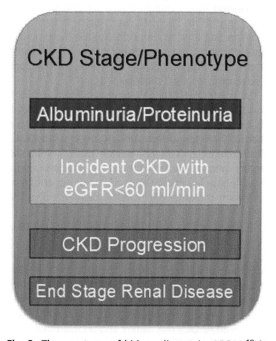
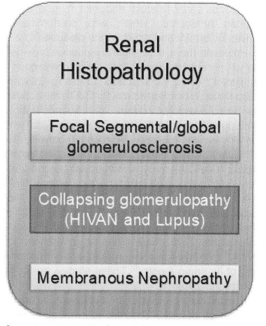

Fig. 2. The spectrum of kidney disease in *APOL1*.[19] (*Data from* Kopp JB, Rosenberg AZ. One actor, many roles: histopathologies associated with APOL1 genetic variants. Adv Anat Pathol 2019;26(3):215–9.)

controversial. Again, it is well known that African Americans are known to have a higher incidence of CVD compared with European Americans.[24] Although the overall rate of death attributable to CVD has decreased from 2003 to 2013 by 28.8%, the rates have been much higher in African American men compared with white men (356 vs 270 per 100,000 Americans, respectively).[25] Thus ethnic-specific genetic factors contribute, and APOL1 might play a role.

Initial evidence for this association was found in 2014. Ito and colleagues[26] used longitudinal clinical and APOL1 genotype data from the Jackson Heart Study (1959 AAs) and found that there was a 2-fold increased risk for CVD events in patients with APOL1 high-risk genotype, even after correcting for both traditional CVD risk factors and CKD. This was replicated with the Women's Health Initiative cohort, which found an increased risk in APOL1 high-risk genotype. Another study analyzing the Cardiovascular Heart Study (CHS), which showed that the risk genotype is associated with the APOL1 genotype, is associated with subclinical atherosclerosis, incident myocardial infarction, and mortality in African Americans >65 years of age.[27] Additional evidence was provided by an autopsy study that showed that the risk genotype was associated with an early age of cardiovascular death independent of nephrosclerosis.[28] Finally, recently in the REGARDS (Reasons for Geographic and Racial Differences in Stroke) cohort, the APOL1 high-risk genotype was found to be associated with a greater risk of composite cardiovascular endpoint in nondiabetic African Americans, which was predominantly driven by stroke and small vessel disease.[29]

However, there is conflicting evidence provided by 2 recent studies. Chen and colleagues[30] analyzed the AASK cohort and found no significant association for increased risk for CVD events, such as cardiovascular death or hospitalization, although there may be a weak association with cardiovascular mortality. A recent analysis, the Coronary Artery Risk Development in Young Adults (CARDIA) study, showed that coronary artery calcification and carotid artery intimal thickness and left ventricular hypertrophy did not differ according to APOL1 genotype.[31] Finally, in the post hoc analysis of Systolic Blood Pressure Intervention Trial, there were no differences by APOL1 genotype in the composite outcome or in any of its components.[32] These studies are summarized in **Table 1**.

So how do we interpret the conflicting evidence from these studies? Differences in study design, study populations, and the handling of confounding data of kidney function may potentially account for these differing conclusions. In addition, survival bias in these cohorts may play a major role in these discrepant findings. Thus, the issue of CVD and APOL1 remains very much an open question and should be addressed by longitudinal, carefully designed studies, and mechanistic experiments.

APOL1 AND HYPERTENSION: THE PLOT THICKENS FURTHER

Essential hypertension is a multifactorial disorder, and significant ethnic differences exist in incidence and prevalence. African Americans with either treated or untreated hypertension have significantly higher mean systolic blood pressure than non-Hispanic white adults.[33] Hypertension is diagnosed earlier in life and at higher frequencies in African Americans compared with other ethnicities.[34] Hypertension is known to be highly heritable. Thus, African Americans not only have environmental and socioeconomic factors contributing to hypertension, but genetics also plays a role in this disparity.[35]

There have been 2 studies looking at blood pressure, APOL1, and hypertension. Using genetic data linked to electronic medical record phenotypic data from several biobanks in the Electronic Medical Records and Genomics (eMERGE) Network for 10,000 individuals, a study found that the APOL1 high-risk genotype was associated with earlier onset of hypertension and increased blood pressure after adjusting for kidney function. Increased blood pressure was evident in individuals aged 20 to 29 years, well before kidney function decline started. Importantly, the increment in blood pressure was linked to per risk variant, rather than the risk genotype. These associations replicated across 3 biobanks.[36]

In contrast to these findings, Chen and colleagues[37] conducted a longitudinal study over 25 years with the CARDIA cohort of 1330 black patients. They found that African American patients had overall significant higher blood pressures than whites. However, they were unable to find a statistically significant association of hypertension between patients with APOL1 high risk and low risk.

These findings need to be interpreted in light of their differences in the studies. The eMERGE cross-sectional study with a large cohort, comprising several age groups of over 9000 participants, had a large number of blood pressure measurements per participant. Thus, it was powered to detect weaker associations of blood pressure with APOL1 risk alleles and showed that each copy of the APOL1 risk variant was associated with an increment in systolic blood pressure.

Table 1
Studies of APOL1 association with CVD

Study Year	Cohort	N	Clinical Outcome	Adjusted Effect Size (CI 95%)	Overall Conclusion	References
2014	Jackson Heart Study	1959	Incident CVD	OR 2.17 (1.34–3.48)	*APOL1* high-risk genotype associated with higher atherosclerotic CVD risk	Ito et al,[26] 2014
	Women's Health Initiative	749		OR 1.98 (1.17–3.31)		
2016	CHS	798	Incident CVD	HR 1.8 (1.1–3.0)	*APOL1* high-risk genotype associated with subclinical atherosclerosis, incident myocardial infarction, and mortality in older African Americans	Mukamal et al,[27] 2016
2017	AASK	693	CVD event	HR 1.16 (0.77–1.76)	*APOL1* high-risk genotype not associated with an overall risk for CVD in AA with hypertension-attributed CKD	Chen et al,[30] 2017
2017	SPRINT	2571	CVD	HR 1.2 (0.76–1.92)	*APOL1* high-risk genotype not associated with incident CVD in high-risk hypertensive patients	Freedman et al,[32] 2017
2017	Autopsy data	298	CAD	OR 1.33 (1.09–1.64)	*APOL1* high-risk genotype are associated with earlier age deaths due to coronary artery disease and cardiomyopathy	Hughson et al,[28] 2018
2018	CARDIA	1315	Prevalence coronary artery calcification LV hypertrophy	RR 1.04 (0.70–1.54) RR 0.96 (0.70–1.33)	*APOL1* high-risk genotype is not associated with subclinical atherosclerotic disease or LVH	Gutiérrez et al,[31] 2018
2018	REGARDS	10,605	Incident CVD	HR 1.67 (1.12–2.47)	*APOL1* high-risk genotype is associated with CVD events in community-dwelling AAs	Gutiérrez et al,[29] 2018

Abbreviations: AA, African American; AASK, African American Study of Kidney; CARDIA, The Coronary Artery Risk Development in Young Adults (CARDIA) study; CHS, cardiovascular health study; CVD, cardiovascular disease; HR, hazard ratio; OR, odds ratio; REGARDS, Reasons for geographic and racial differences in stroke study; SPRINT, Systolic Blood Pressure Intervention Trial.

However, all participants were all hospital-based and may have had higher comorbid disease and did not include ambulatory blood pressure measurements. Although the study by Chen and colleagues was smaller, it was longitudinal and in an observational cohort. Because the study was also underpowered to detect associations of *APOL1* risk alleles with blood pressure, it thus may require a much larger sample size, especially as the differences in blood pressure were very small for each risk variant. In addition, there was no replication cohort, which is important for studies of associations between genotype and phenotype.

HYPERTENSION, KIDNEY DISEASE AND *APOL1*: INEXTRICABLY CONNECTED?

The relationship between hypertension and CKD is complicated because they perpetuate each other. The cause of hypertensive renal disease is multifactorial. Long-term uncontrolled hypertension causes arteriolar nephrosclerosis, leading to glomerular ischemia. As renal function declines, hypertension usually worsens. Limited salt excretion, salt sensitivity, and extracellular fluid volume expansion are key mechanisms for poor blood pressure control in patients with CKD. These patients also have increased oxidative stress and worse atherosclerotic disease. Hypertension accelerates kidney disease with a vicious cycle of renin-angiotensin-aldosterone system activation, systemic vasoconstriction, and glomerular hypertension.[38]

The association of *APOL1* and hypertension is not completely understood. Individuals with risk variants do have higher blood pressure and higher risk of CKD. Does the kidney disease in these patients cause the higher blood pressure or does the higher blood pressure cause the kidney disease, or are these 2 entities caused by separate mechanisms? Because not everyone with *APOL1* high-risk variants develops kidney disease, there may also be a question of a "second hit" that triggers CKD and progression (**Fig. 3**).[39]

WHAT DOES THE FUTURE HOLD FOR *APOL1*?

APOL1 risk variants are common in persons of African ancestry (including African Americans and Hispanic Americans) and are one of the most powerful disease variants identified to date in terms of frequency and effect size for kidney disease. This is an important discovery for nephrology and has helped further our understanding of disparities. There are efforts to incorporate genetic testing in routine clinical settings, including in pretransplant evaluation and as a therapeutic target.[40,41]

The association of *APOL1* with other linked diseases, such as CVD and hypertension, is still controversial. The evidence from epidemiologic and observational studies is conflicting and there is, as yet, no mechanistic evidence. However, *APOL1* is broadly expressed in human tissues, raising the question of whether the *APOL1* risk allele toxicity is restricted to kidney diseases. In addition, genetic variants usually exhibit

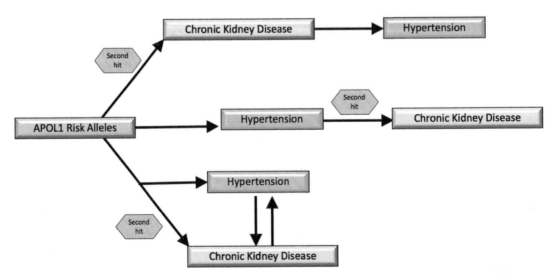

Fig. 3. The possible relationships between *APOL1* risk alleles, CKD, and hypertension. *APOL1* risk alleles cause CKD causing hypertension. (*Data from* Nadkarni GN, Coca SG. APOL1 and blood pressure changes in young adults. Kidney Int 2017;92(4):793–5.)

pleiotropy, which is association with many pheno-types.[42] In addition, it has been proposed that there may be a possible unifying mechanism of endothelial dysfunction leading to both kidney disease and CVD.[43] However, definitive answers are lacking, and thus the association with CVD and hypertension should still be considered an open question.

Regardless, the role of *APOL1* genetic testing in clinical medicine needs to be studied. Clinical trials such as the Genetic Testing to Understand and Address Renal Disease Disparities are ongoing, in which patients are randomized to undergo genotyping for the *APOL1* risk variants with clinical decision support or to usual care.[44] These studies are essential to understanding the role that testing will play in clinical outcomes, and ultimately what the benefit to patients is, the ultimate goal of translational research.

REFERENCES

1. Kruzel-Davila E, Wasser WG, Skorecki K. APOL1 nephropathy: a population genetics and evolutionary medicine detective story. Semin Nephrol 2017; 37(6):490–507.
2. Pérez-Morga D, Vanhollebeke B, Paturiaux-Hanocq F, et al. Apolipoprotein L-I promotes trypanosome lysis by forming pores in lysosomal membranes. Science 2005;309(5733):469–72.
3. Friedman DJ, Pollak MR. Genetics of kidney failure and the evolving story of APOL1. J Clin Invest 2011;121(9):3367–74.
4. Kao WHL, Klag MJ, Meoni LA, et al. MYH9 is associated with nondiabetic end-stage renal disease in African Americans. Nat Genet 2008;40(10):1185–92.
5. Genovese G, Friedman DJ, Ross MD, et al. Association of trypanolytic ApoL1 variants with kidney disease in African Americans. Science 2010; 329(5993):841–5.
6. Limou S, Nelson GW, Kopp JB, et al. APOL1 kidney risk alleles: population genetics and disease associations. Adv Chronic Kidney Dis 2014;21(5):426–33.
7. Behar DM, Kedem E, Rosset S, et al. Absence of APOL1 risk variants protects against HIV-associated nephropathy in the Ethiopian population. Am J Nephrol 2011;34(5):452–9.
8. Matsha TE, Kengne AP, Masconi KL, et al. APOL1 genetic variants, chronic kidney diseases and hypertension in mixed ancestry South Africans. BMC Genet 2015;16(1):69.
9. Nadkarni G, Gignoux C, Sorokin E, et al. Worldwide frequencies of APOL1 renal risk variants. N Engl J Med 2018;379(26):2571–2.
10. Udler MS, Nadkarni GN, Belbin G, et al. Effect of genetic African ancestry on eGFR and kidney disease. J Am Soc Nephrol 2015;26(7):1682–92.
11. McClellan W, Warnock DG, McClure L, et al. Racial differences in the prevalence of chronic kidney disease among participants in the reasons for geographic and racial differences in stroke (REGARDS) cohort study. J Am Soc Nephrol 2006; 17(6):1710–5.
12. Choi AI, Rodriguez RA, Bacchetti P, et al. White/black racial differences in risk of end-stage renal disease and death. Am J Med 2009;122(7):672–8.
13. Hsu C-Y, Lin F, Vittinghoff E, et al. Racial differences in the progression from chronic renal insufficiency to end-stage renal disease in the United States. J Am Soc Nephrol 2003;14(11):2902–7.
14. Kopp JB, Nelson GW, Sampath K, et al. APOL1 genetic variants in focal segmental glomerulosclerosis and HIV-associated nephropathy. J Am Soc Nephrol 2011;22(11):2129–37.
15. Foster MC, Coresh J, Fornage M, et al. APOL1 variants associate with increased risk of CKD among African Americans. J Am Soc Nephrol 2013;24(9): 1484–91.
16. Tzur S, Rosset S, Skorecki K, et al. APOL1 allelic variants are associated with lower age of dialysis initiation and thereby increased dialysis vintage in African and Hispanic Americans with non-diabetic end-stage kidney disease. Nephrol Dial Transplant 2012;27(4):1498–505.
17. Kanji Z, Powe CE, Wenger JB, et al. Genetic variation in APOL1 associates with younger age at hemodialysis initiation. J Am Soc Nephrol 2011;22(11): 2091–7.
18. Parsa A, Kao WHL, Xie D, et al. APOL1 risk variants, race, and progression of chronic kidney disease. N Engl J Med 2013;369(23):2183–96.
19. Kopp JB, Rosenberg AZ. One actor, many roles: histopathologies associated with APOL1 genetic variants. Adv Anat Pathol 2019;26(3):215–9.
20. Granado D, Müller D, Krausel V, et al. Intracellular APOL1 risk variants cause cytotoxicity accompanied by energy depletion. J Am Soc Nephrol 2017; 28(11):3227–38.
21. Beckerman P, Bi-Karchin J, Park ASD, et al. Transgenic expression of human APOL1 risk variants in podocytes induces kidney disease in mice. Nat Med 2017;23(4):429–38.
22. Ma L, Chou JW, Snipes JA, et al. APOL1 renal-risk variants induce mitochondrial dysfunction. J Am Soc Nephrol 2017;28(4):1093–105.
23. Hayek SS, Koh KH, Grams ME, et al. A tripartite complex of suPAR, APOL1 risk variants and αvβ3 integrin on podocytes mediates chronic kidney disease. Nat Med 2017;23(8):945–53.
24. Pool LR, Ning H, Lloyd-Jones DM, et al. Trends in racial/ethnic disparities in cardiovascular health among US adults from 1999-2012. J Am Heart Assoc 2017;6. https://doi.org/10.1161/JAHA.117.006027.

25. Benjamin EJ, Virani SS, Callaway CW, et al. Heart disease and stroke statistics-2018 update: a report from the American Heart Association. Circulation 2018;137(12):e67–492.

26. Ito K, Bick AG, Flannick J, et al. Increased burden of cardiovascular disease in carriers of APOL1 genetic variants. Circ Res 2014;114(5):845–50.

27. Mukamal KJ, Tremaglio J, Friedman DJ, et al. APOL1 genotype, kidney and cardiovascular disease, and death in older adults. Arterioscler Thromb Vasc Biol 2016;36(2):398–403.

28. Hughson MD, Hoy WE, Mott SA, et al. APOL1 risk variants independently associated with early cardiovascular disease death. Kidney Int Rep 2018;3(1):89–98.

29. Gutiérrez OM, Irvin MR, Chaudhary NS, et al. APOL1 nephropathy risk variants and incident cardiovascular disease events in community-dwelling black adults. Circ Genom Precis Med 2018;11(6):e002098.

30. Chen TK, Appel LJ, Grams ME, et al. APOL1 risk variants and cardiovascular disease: results from the AASK (African American study of kidney disease and hypertension). Arterioscler Thromb Vasc Biol 2017;37(9):1765–9.

31. Gutiérrez OM, Limou S, Lin F, et al. APOL1 nephropathy risk variants do not associate with subclinical atherosclerosis or left ventricular mass in middle-aged black adults. Kidney Int 2018;93(3):727–32.

32. Freedman BI, Rocco MV, Bates JT, et al. APOL1 renal-risk variants do not associate with incident cardiovascular disease or mortality in the Systolic Blood Pressure Intervention Trial. Kidney Int Rep 2017;2(4):713–20.

33. Wright JD, Hughes JP, Ostchega Y, et al. Mean systolic and diastolic blood pressure in adults aged 18 and over in the United States, 2001-2008. Natl Health Stat Report 2011;(35):1–22, 24.

34. Hajjar I, Kotchen TA. Trends in prevalence, awareness, treatment, and control of hypertension in the United States, 1988-2000. JAMA 2003;290(2):199–206.

35. Waken RJ, de Las Fuentes L, Rao DC. A review of the genetics of hypertension with a focus on gene-environment interactions. Curr Hypertens Rep 2017;19(3):23.

36. Nadkarni GN, Galarneau G, Ellis SB, et al. Apolipoprotein L1 variants and blood pressure traits in African Americans. J Am Coll Cardiol 2017;69(12):1564–74.

37. Chen TK, Estrella MM, Vittinghoff E, et al. APOL1 genetic variants are not associated with longitudinal blood pressure in young black adults. Kidney Int 2017;92(4):964–71.

38. Judd E, Calhoun DA. Management of hypertension in CKD: beyond the guidelines. Adv Chronic Kidney Dis 2015;22(2):116–22.

39. Nadkarni GN, Coca SG. APOL1 and blood pressure changes in young adults. Kidney Int 2017;92(4):793–5.

40. Freedman BI, Moxey-Mims M. The APOL1 long-term kidney transplantation outcomes network-APOLLO. Clin J Am Soc Nephrol 2018;13(6):940–2.

41. Heymann J, Winkler CA, Hoek M, et al. Therapeutics for APOL1 nephropathies: putting out the fire in the podocyte. Nephrol Dial Transplant 2017;32(suppl_1):i65–70.

42. The landscape of pervasive horizontal pleiotropy in human genetic variation is driven by extreme polygenicity of human traits and diseases | bioRxiv [Internet]. Available at: https://www.biorxiv.org/content/10.1101/311332v1. Accessed March 12, 2019.

43. Estrella MM, Parekh RS. The expanding role of APOL1 risk in chronic kidney disease and cardiovascular disease. Semin Nephrol 2017;37(6):520–9.

44. Horowitz CR, Abul-Husn NS, Ellis S, et al. Determining the effects and challenges of incorporating genetic testing into primary care management of hypertensive patients with African ancestry. Contemp Clin Trials 2016;47:101–8.

Novel Antidiabetic Therapies and Cardiovascular Risk Reduction
The Role of the Noninferiority Trial

Jillian Thompson, DO[a], Sydney Schacht, DO[a],
Florence Rothenberg, MS, MD[a,b],*

KEYWORDS

- Empagliflozin • Liraglutide • Cardiovascular risk • Mortality • Noninferiority trial

KEY POINTS

- Two large noninferiority trials demonstrated that empagliflozin and liraglutide are associated with reduced cardiovascular composite outcomes in patients with type 2 diabetes mellitus (T2DM), and who are at risk for atherosclerotic events.
- Both drugs were effective in slowing progression of renal dysfunction, and may be the first drugs to impact cardiorenal syndrome.
- The effects of diet, exercise, and smoking cessation were not reported in these trials; whether the benefit of these medications persists with lifestyle improvement is unclear.
- Additional trials are needed to confirm these results, and to determine whether they can be generalized to women, nonwhite patients, lower doses of medication, and lower-risk patients.
- Adverse events and risks were low; therefore, *at the very least*, nonendocrinologists should consider referring their patients with T2DM to endocrinologists to determine if they would benefit. A streamlined team-approach to management of these patients must be considered.

INTRODUCTION

It is well established that type 2 diabetes (T2DM) is associated with increased risk of mortality due to cardiovascular and microvascular disease.[1] Several classes of medications approved for treatment of T2DM have proven successful in reducing both hemoglobin A1c (HgA1c) and microvascular complications.[2,3] Although HgA1c is clearly a marker for cardiovascular outcomes,[4] the cardiovascular benefit from aggressive lowering of the HgA1c is less clear.[5] Several novel agents have recently been developed to reduce blood glucose in patients with T2DM. In part because of the relationship between T2DM and cardiovascular events, the Food and Drug Administration (FDA) in 2008 issued guidelines to pharmaceutical companies requiring that new diabetes drugs demonstrate cardiovascular safety[6] in cardiovascular outcomes trials.

Many of these trials have been completed in the past few years, evaluating drugs from several different classes, including DPP-4 inhibitors, GLP-1 agonists, and SGLT2 inhibitors. Two of these agents, empagliflozin (SGLT-2 inhibitor) and liraglutide (GLP-1 agonist), were the first

Disclosure Statement: The authors have nothing to disclose.
[a] Department of Internal Medicine, University of Cincinnati Medical Center, University of Cincinnati, 51 Goodman Drive, Cincinnati, OH 45267, USA; [b] University of Cincinnati, VAMC Cincinnati, 3200 Vine Street, Cincinnati, OH 45267, USA
* Corresponding author. VAMC Cincinnati, 3200 Vine Street ML111C, Cincinnati, OH 45267.
E-mail address: florence.rothenberg@uc.edu

Cardiol Clin 37 (2019) 335–343
https://doi.org/10.1016/j.ccl.2019.04.007
0733-8651/19/Published by Elsevier Inc.

agents reported to show superiority in cardiovascular and renal outcomes when added to standard of care. This review focuses on critical evaluation of the trials EMPA-REG OUTCOMES,[7] which examined the impact of empagliflozin on cardiovascular safety, and LEADER,[8] which examined the impact of liraglutide on cardiovascular safety. The first goal of this review was to show how the noninferiority trial design is suited to address the question of cardiovascular safety of these agents. The second goal was to develop a portrait of the patients who should be considered for use of these agents. Ultimately, it is our hope that this review will provide the reader with a foundation on which to understand the noninferiority trial in general, and how these 2 trials in particular provide snapshots of patients who may benefit from these new interventions. For more detailed information on how to use these agents, the reader may be referred to the 2018 American College of Cardiology Expert Consensus[2] and the Endocrine Society guidelines.[3]

TRIAL DESIGN BASICS

We are intuitively familiar with superiority studies in which 2 treatments are compared, the goal of which is to determine if a new treatment is associated with benefits over an accepted treatment. The gold standard for such decision making is the randomized, double-blind, placebo-controlled trial (RCT), in which patients who are at risk for the outcome being investigated (eg, cardiovascular events, improved HgA1c, blood pressure goals) are randomly placed into one group (standard of care, placebo, active accepted therapy) or the other (new treatment).

Let us review these basic components of a "gold standard" clinical trial:

1. Randomization of patients: investigators generate a protocol before study enrollment whereby successive patients who qualify to be enrolled in a trial are randomly selected to be in one group or the other. Randomization reduces the possibility that by chance we have selected a population of patients who may do better (or worse) with the study treatment. Adequate randomization should also have the effect of creating 2 similar populations with respect to risk factors and demographics of interest. The more rigorous the randomization, the less bias (any departure from the truth) will be introduced into the study conclusions.
2. Double-blind: Neither the investigators nor the patients know into which group the patient has been randomized. This also minimizes

potential bias of the study conclusions, as knowledge of the treatment may subtly influence behavior that could change the outcome of a trial. The less the patient or the investigator knows about the treatment arm of the study, the less likely this knowledge will impact behavior.
3. Placebo controls: A placebo should be a physiologically inert but otherwise identical intervention. In theory, this should be the most vigorous comparison possible: an active intervention versus an identical yet inactive intervention. Some trialists believe that a placebo comparator is necessary in all clinical trials, even when comparing a new intervention with an active but accepted intervention. Use of a placebo may be considered unethical, however, particularly when the accepted treatment reduces mortality in an otherwise potentially fatal illness. For this reason, many investigations compare a new treatment with an active and accepted therapy and do not include a placebo control group.

Trialists adhere to these predefined trial components to minimize bias, or any feature of a trial that may cause a departure from the truth. The truth, in this case, is knowing whether our new intervention will increase, decrease, or have no effect on cardiovascular events. With respect to this review, we want to know whether EMPA-REG OUTCOMES[7] (EMPA-REG) and LEADER[8] trials truly did show that empagliflozin and/or liraglutide were safe with respect to cardiovascular events.

WHO SHOULD BE INCLUDED IN THIS CLINICAL TRIAL?

Patients should be considered for inclusion in a trial if they are *at risk for* the outcome we are attempting to prevent, and these risks are defined by *inclusion criteria*. In contrast, patients who may be harmed by the intervention are defined by *exclusion criteria*. Exclusion criteria are determined from adverse events that occur in preclinical trials of humans and animal studies. Inclusion and exclusion criteria are specified in the trial protocol before the trial begins, in contrast to the *demographics* of a study, which describe the patients who completed the trial. This discussion focuses on EMPA-REG and LEADER trial *major* inclusion and exclusion criteria only. Detailed inclusion and exclusion criteria can be found in the published protocols.[9,10]

EMPA-REG specifically included only patients with T2DM *with a known history of* cardiovascular disease, and therefore at highest risk for future cardiovascular events. In contrast, the LEADER trial had 2 separate subgroups of patients: older (≥60 years old) patients with T2DM who had at least 1 additional risk factor for cardiovascular events, and younger patients with T2DM (≥50 years old) who had known cardiovascular disease. This difference may have diluted the impact of the clinical effect observed for liraglutide, as will be described later.

In both trials, a primary exclusion criterion was presence of type 1 diabetes mellitus (T1DM), primarily because insulin replacement is known to prevent morbidity and mortality in patients with T1DM. SGLT2 inhibitors may cause increased risk of diabetic ketoacidosis[11]; however, several studies are under way to assess for this.[12]

Preclinical investigations of empagliflozin found that renal dysfunction increases the likelihood of hypotension and urinary tract infections. Therefore, patients with estimated glomerular filtration rate (eGFR) less than 30 mL/min per 1.73 m^2 (modification of diet in renal disease equation) were excluded from EMPA-REG. Liraglutide in contrast was rarely observed to cause alterations in renal function; patients with eGFR less than 30 mL/min per 1.73 m^2 were not excluded, but despite this were still only a small fraction of patients enrolled (approximately 2.5%) in LEADER.

Preclinical trials of liraglutide found an increased incidence of multiple endocrine neoplasia type 2 and medullary thyroid carcinoma; therefore, patients who had a personal or family history of these cancers were excluded. Empagliflozin, on the other hand, was not associated with particular cancers in preclinical trials, and only a general exclusion of patients experiencing malignancies that could confound mortality outcomes were excluded from this trial.

Demographics, on the other hand, provide a snapshot of all the patients who were enrolled in the trial. The demographics (or patient characteristics) section is often in the form of a large table in which the number of patients in the placebo group with characteristics of interest are compared with the number of patients in the active comparator arm. Detailed demographics are typically found in supplementary appendices published as a link with the original report. It is often the goal of the investigators to include as wide a variety of patients as possible. Review of the demographics section shows how diverse the patient population is or is not, and allows comparison of the patients who were enrolled in the treatment and placebo arms.

The demographics section should address whether there was a statistically significant difference in the subgroups that might influence outcomes. *Knowing the inclusion and exclusion criteria, as well as the demographics, allows the clinician to create a profile of the patient who might benefit from a new drug.*

WHAT IS THE PURPOSE OF A NONINFERIORITY TRIAL?

As noted in the Introduction, the FDA recommended in 2008 that new treatments for T2DM had to prove cardiovascular safety. The question, therefore, is not whether one agent is better than placebo or standard of care, but whether the new medications cause excess cardiovascular harm. The respective goals of EMPA-REG and LEADER, then, were to show that empagliflozin and liraglutide were not unacceptably worse than accepted therapy with regard to cardiovascular outcomes.

HOW DO NONINFERIORITY TRIALS WORK?

Similar to superiority trials, noninferiority trials also should be randomized, controlled, and blinded to minimize bias. To establish if empagliflozin and liraglutide were not "unacceptably worse" with respect to cardiovascular outcomes, investigators study the literature to determine how many cardiovascular events could be expected in the standard-of-care groups. This becomes the "point estimate" to which the new agents, empagliflozin and liraglutide, will be compared (**Fig. 1**, solid vertical line labeled "Point Estimate for Standard Therapy").

Trialists and statisticians use data from published trials, discussion, and consensus to determine a "noninferiority margin," or a range of cardiovascular events that the trialists consider not "unacceptably worse" than standard therapy (see **Fig. 1**, dashed vertical line). The difference between the standard-of-care point estimate for cardiovascular events and the proposed difference in cardiovascular events that would be "not unacceptably worse" is called the noninferiority margin, or delta (Δ). Both EMPA-REG OUTCOME and LEADER trials selected a margin of 1.3[7,8] (**Table 1**).

If the point estimate and confidence interval of the new treatment (black circle and brackets) fall above the noninferiority margin (Δ) on the side favoring active treatment (liraglutide or empagliflozin), the new treatment may be considered "noninferior" (A and B). If the goal of the trial is to show noninferiority, the investigators could conclude a positive outcome if the result was either A or B, and the drug would be considered noninferior. Alternatively, the point estimate and

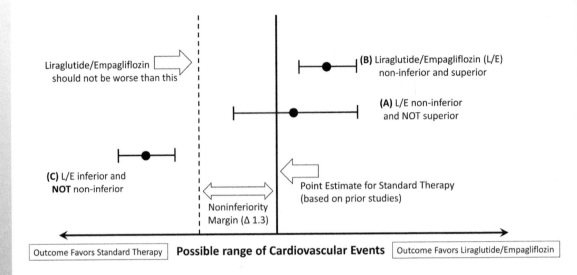

Fig. 1. Select potential outcomes for noninferiority trial of liraglutide/empagliflozin (L/E). (*Adapted from* Schumi J, Wittes JT. Through the looking glass: understanding non-inferiority. Trials 2011;12:106; with permission.)

Table 1
Patients included in EMPA-REG and LEADER trials

Characteristics of Patients in EMPA-REG OUTCOMES and LEADER Trials		
	EMPA-REG Outcomes	**LEADER**
Primary outcome	CV death, nonfatal MI, nonfatal stroke (no silent MI)	CV death, nonfatal MI, nonfatal stroke (with silent MI)
Major inclusion criteria	T2DM, HgA1c >7.0% >18 y + established CV disease (prior stroke, MI, PCI, PVD, known CAD)	T2DM, HgA1c >7.0% ≥50 y + CV coexisting OR ≥60 y and 1 CV risk factor
Demographics		
Age	63.2 y (avg)	64 y (avg)
Gender	Male (71%)	Male (64%)
Ethnicity	White (72%)	White (77.5%)
Region	European (41%)	European (35%)
BMI	31 kg/m² (avg)	32.5 kg/m²
HgA1c	8.07% (avg)	8.7% (avg)
Duration of T2DM diagnosis	10 y (57%)	12.8 y (avg)
On metformin	74%	76%
Renal function	eGFR 60–90 mL/min per 1.73 m² (52%)	eGFR 60–90 mL/min per 1.73 m² (41%)
Positive interaction statistics	Patients with HgA1c <8.5% favored empagliflozin	Patients ≥50 and known CV disease and those with eGFR 30–60 mL/min per 1.73 m² favored liraglutide

Inclusion criteria were determined before the trial, whereas demographics were collected after the trial. The demographics describe most patients who were represented in the trial. Positive interaction statistics identifies predetermined groups where there was a significant difference observed in benefit between those with and without the particular characteristic as indicated.

Abbreviations: avg, average; BMI, body mass index; CAD, coronary artery disease; CV, cardiovascular; eGFR, estimated glomerular filtration rate; HgA1c, hemoglobin A1c; MI, myocardial infarction; PCI, percutaneous intervention; PVD, peripheral vascular disease; T2DM, type 2 diabetes mellitus.

confidence intervals for the new drug may fall below the noninferiority margin (C), and the new drug would be considered both inferior and NOT noninferior.

It can be appropriate to design a clinical trial to show a new treatment is superior in a noninferiority trial, but only *after* noninferiority has been demonstrated, whereby margins and outcome goals have been determined and agreed on before patient enrollment begins. In contrast, if a new drug is tested against standard therapy in a superiority trial but is shown to be effective but not superior, it is inappropriate to say the new drug is noninferior. This is because the statistical tools for superiority and noninferiority trial are different, and outcome goals (eg, noninferiority margin, point estimates for comparison) must be agreed on before a trial is initiated.

POTENTIAL PROBLEMS WITH THE NONINFERIORITY DESIGN

Noninferiority studies may be rewarded by poor performance.[13] Let us say a noninferiority study of Gonzogliptin (made-up drug) fails to properly randomize patients. Unbeknownst to the investigators, the active drug arm has fewer patients who would benefit from the drug. This might occur if, for example, the investigators decide to enroll every other patient into one or the other study group rather than using a more rigorous randomization method. By chance, the Gonzogliptin group has fewer patients at risk for the outcome. Having fewer patients at risk for the outcome makes it look like Gonzogliptin is not working, when in fact there are simply fewer patients who would have benefited in the Gonzogliptin arm. As a result, the study drug is shown to be of no benefit, where in reality Gonzogliptin is beneficial. Because the goal of the study, however, is to show that Gonzogliptin is "not unacceptably worse than" current treatment, this noninferiority trial appears to be successful. Poor study design, therefore, introduced bias that obscured the truth in a way that results in a "positive" noninferiority trial. Gonzogliptin was shown to be noninferior, when in reality it is a superior intervention compared with standard therapy. This underscores the necessity for rigorous, prospective trial design.

Noninferiority studies like the Gonzogliptin trial that fail to demonstrate a difference when there truly is one, are said to lack "assay sensitivity." Assay sensitivity is defined as "the ability of a clinical trial to distinguish between an effective and ineffective treatment."[14] If a trial is designed to show superiority and is then definitive in showing the new drug is effective or ineffective, the study

has assay sensitivity. Including a placebo control is another way to increase assay sensitivity, particularly if superiority of the new drug is also demonstrated. Both EMPA-REG and LEADER were designed to show superiority (after noninferiority was demonstrated), and a placebo control was used. Use of a placebo was considered ethical here, as it was not yet known that both agents had a significant impact on cardiovascular mortality. If empagliflozin or liraglutide were to demonstrate that they are superior to a placebo control, then the clinical trial will have distinguished "between an effective and ineffective treatment."

In summary, the EMPA-REG OUTCOMES and LEADER trials were both carefully, prospectively designed randomized, placebo-controlled, double-blinded, noninferiority studies that were designed to demonstrate superiority, after noninferiority was demonstrated, and therefore had acceptable assay sensitivity. Both trials are discussed with respect to the target population (a general description of who would likely benefit from the drug), the outcomes, and limitations.

EMPAGLIFLOZIN: EMPA-REG TRIAL

Empagliflozin is an SGLT-2 inhibitor and works by inhibiting the reabsorption of both glucose and sodium in the proximal tubules, and leads to increased urinary excretion of sodium and glucose. The EMPA-REG OUTCOME trial was published in 2015 and randomized 7020 patients to receiving either empagliflozin (10 mg or 25 mg daily) or placebo, with median follow-up time of 3.1 years. The investigators hypothesized that empagliflozin would be noninferior to placebo with regard to the primary composite outcome of death from cardiovascular causes, nonfatal myocardial infarction (MI), or nonfatal stroke.

The major *inclusion criteria* were patients with T2DM and established cardiovascular disease, body mass index (BMI) less than 45, and hemoglobin A1c of at least 7.0%. *Major exclusion criteria* included patients with hemoglobin A1c greater than 10.0% and eGFR less than 30 mL/min per 1.73 m^2.

Most patients enrolled in the trial (the *demographics* of the study population) were white (~72%), male (~71%), and European (~41%), with glycated hemoglobin of ~8.07%, BMI ~31, and eGFR between 60 and 90 mL/min per 1.73 m^2 (~52%). Review of the detailed demographics table (in the supplementary appendix) showed that there were no significant baseline differences between both empagliflozin groups and patients randomized to placebo. Once the study was under way, however, more patients in the placebo group were started on angiotensin-converting enzyme (ACE) inhibitors (27.4 vs 23.6), diuretics (22.7 vs 16.2), beta-blockers (18 vs 15.9), calcium channel blockers (18.3 vs 12.6), and mineralocorticoid receptor antagonists (4.7 vs 2.9).

The main finding of EMPA-REG was that among the *pooled treatment groups*, empagliflozin treatment resulted in *reduction of the primary composite outcome* of cardiovascular deaths, nonfatal MI, and nonfatal stroke, as well as a significant reduction in hospitalizations for heart failure (hazard ratio 0.86, 95.02% confidence interval [CI] 0.74–0.99; $P<.001$ for noninferiority and $P = .04$ for superiority). This result appeared to have been driven by a significantly lower risk of cardiovascular death, in which survival curves were found to separate very early after initiation of treatment. This result was despite only a modest reduction in glycated hemoglobin (−0.42% points and −0.47% points in the 10 mg and 25 mg groups, respectively).

The trial was designed to assess for differences in a *composite* outcome, not the individual components. In a published letter,[15] the investigators make a reasonable argument as to why it may be acceptable to conclude benefits for cardiovascular mortality alone. They point out that the 38% reduction in cardiovascular mortality was robust across many variables, and remained significant despite several different sensitivity analyses. These findings led to an unprecedented FDA approval for empagliflozin in the reduction in cardiovascular death, despite that this was not an explicit part of the confirmatory testing hierarchy.

Examination of predetermined subgroups is common in clinical trials, primarily to determine whether any groups stand out with respect to harm or benefit. EMPA-REG subgroup analyses showed a statistically significant benefit in patients who were ≤65 years, or with glycated hemoglobin ≤8.5%. Statistical significance here refers to interaction statistics, which are designed to determine if a particular variable has a significant impact on the outcome that is being measured. Although statistically significant, the number of patients in subgroup analyses are not sufficient to make definitive conclusions, and these findings must be confirmed with appropriately designed studies.

A prespecified analysis of the 7020 patients enrolled in EMPA-REG was designed to study effects of empagliflozin on progression of renal disease in these patients with T2DM and cardiovascular disease.[16] New or progressing nephropathy had a significant relative risk reduction of 39%, progression to microalbuminuria a relative risk reduction of 38%, doubling of creatinine relative

risk reduction of 44%, and initiation of renal replacement therapy relative risk reduction of 44%, with 3 deaths from renal disease in the empagliflozin group and none in the placebo group. Interestingly, there was an initial decrease in eGFR with initiation of empagliflozin similar to that seen with ACE inhibitors. Over time, eGFR worsened to a greater degree in the placebo group. When empagliflozin was discontinued, the eGFR returned to near normal in the empagliflozin group, but remained lower in the placebo group. In patients with renal disease at the start of the trial, empagliflozin reduced cardiovascular death, all-cause mortality, and all-cause hospitalization as compared with placebo, independent of renal function.[17]

LIRAGLUTIDE: LEADER TRIAL

Liraglutide is a glucagonlike peptide-1 (GLP-1) receptor agonist, and an injectable medication in contrast to empagliflozin. GLP-1 agonists are incretin mimetics and work by stimulating insulin release from the pancreatic beta cells in response to glucose.[18] Published in 2016, the LEADER trial randomized 9340 patients to receive either daily liraglutide or placebo with median follow-up time of 3.8 years. The investigators hypothesized that liraglutide would be noninferior to placebo with regard to the primary composite outcome: first occurrence of cardiovascular mortality, nonfatal MI, or nonfatal stroke.

Like EMPA-REG, *major inclusion criteria* were patients with T2DM with hemoglobin A1c >7.0%; in contrast, however, patients could be either ≥50 years old with at least 1 cardiovascular *coexisting condition*, or ≥60 years with at least 1 cardiovascular risk factor. *Major exclusion criteria* included presence of T1DM, on rapid-acting insulin, pramlintide, GLP-1 receptor agonists or dipeptidyl peptidase 4 (DPP-4) agonists, or if they had a familial or personal history of multiple endocrine neoplasia (MEN) type 2 or medullary thyroid cancer.

The demographics for the LEADER trial are similar to patients enrolled in EMPA-REG: most patients enrolled in the LEADER trial were white (~77.5%), European (~35%), male (~64%), aged ~64, BMI ~32.5, and eGFR between 60 and 90 mL/min per 1.73 m^2 (~41%). In contrast to EMPA-REG, in which ~99% of patients had established cardiovascular disease, only 81.7% of patients enrolled in LEADER were similarly high risk. In addition, review of the detailed demographics in the supplementary appendix also reveals that there was a significantly higher proportion of patients treated with beta-blockers in the liraglutide group. A lower-risk population and more patients in the treatment group taking beta-blockers can potentially dilute any benefit observed with liraglutide.

Like the EMPA-REG trial, the LEADER trial demonstrated a reduction in the primary composite outcome for the liraglutide group compared with placebo, primarily driven by reductions in death from cardiovascular causes (hazard ratio 0.78; 95% CI, 0.66–0.93, $P = .007$), and also all-cause mortality (hazard ratio 0.85; 95% CI 0.74–0.97, $P = .02$). Like the EMPA-REG trial, LEADER was a composite outcome for which the study was powered, not the individual component of cardiovascular death. This result is compelling and exploratory, but not confirmatory. In contrast to empagliflozin, liraglutide survival curves began to diverge much later in the 6-month to 12-month period after treatment was initiated. As with empagliflozin, the clinical benefits observed with liraglutide were seen despite only modest reduction in glycated hemoglobin (−0.40% reduction at 36-month prespecified analysis, 95% CI −0.45 to −0.34). The clinical benefits observed, therefore, appear out of proportion to the impact on glycated hemoglobin.

Similar to empagliflozin, a post hoc analysis showed that patients with eGFR less than 60 mL/min per 1.73 m^2 had reduced composite outcome of cardiovascular death, nonfatal stroke, and MI in the liraglutide group, numerically more so than for patients with eGFR $\geq$60.[19] This was also true for the individual component outcomes and all-cause death. Adverse events were no greater in patients with chronic kidney disease than in those with normal renal function.

LIMITATIONS OF LEADER AND EMPA-REG

The cardiovascular mortality benefit in the LEADER trail was only observed in patients outside the United States.[20] This may be because there was a higher percentage of patients with prior cardiovascular disease in European participants.[21] Despite this, the FDA approved liraglutide for its cardiovascular mortality indication, mainly because the risk reduction in the entire cohort was quite large.

In the EMPA-REG trial, statistical significance was observed only for the primary composite outcome when both the 10-mg and 25-mg doses were pooled. Because survival curves were similar for the 10-mg dose and 25-mg dose separately, the investigators concluded that pooling of the groups was reasonable. Cardiovascular outcomes, however, have not been studied for the lower dose group only; this would be necessary to show that the lower dose was effective on its own in an appropriately powered trial.

The impact of lifestyle adherence was not measured in either investigation. The LEADER trial stated that, "at the time of randomization the importance of lifestyle approaches for diabetes management including dietary changes, physical activity, and weight management should be stressed to all subjects," whereas the EMPA-REG trial noted, "male and female patients on diet and exercise regimen who are drug naïve or pretreated with any background therapy" were included. The EMPA-REG trial had a requirement that diet and exercise counseling occur at all follow-up visits, but it was only noted that "local diet recommendations" were used. Success or failure of lifestyle adherence was not measured. In addition, smoking history was collected in both trials, but outcomes based on smoking were not reported. Last, whether the patients were taking metformin was documented (approximately three-quarters of all patients in both trials were taking metformin); however, outcomes with respect to taking metformin were not reported.

Renal findings are clearly important, yet neither study was designed to assess renal outcomes as primary outcomes. Power analyses and the impact of multiple comparisons were not considered for these secondary outcomes. These results should therefore be seen as hypothesis generating and not confirmatory.

DISCUSSION

The LEADER and EMPA-REG OUTCOME trials showed that liraglutide and empagliflozin are noninferior and superior to standard of care with placebo. Patients with T2DM and high risk for cardiovascular events treated with liraglutide or empagliflozin had significantly fewer events for the combined primary outcome of cardiovascular death, nonfatal MI, and nonfatal stroke. Additional benefits were demonstrated with these medications including improved renal outcomes with both liraglutide and empagliflozin, improved systolic blood pressure, weight loss, and a reduction in heart failure hospitalizations with empagliflozin. Although neither study was designed with cardiovascular death as a confirmatory outcome, the robust nature of reduced mortality across subgroups led to an FDA indication for use of these agents to reduce cardiovascular mortality in these at-risk patients.

We do not yet know if there will be a class effect of these agents, yet many studies are currently under way. It should be remembered that most patients enrolled in these studies were already taking metformin, and thus it is unclear if the benefits are due to either liraglutide or empagliflozin alone, or are instead conferred by the combination of these medications with metformin. In addition, patients who benefited had established cardiovascular disease; those with only risk factors for cardiovascular disease may not benefit from these medications. Both trials included a majority of white men; this benefit may not be extrapolated to women or other races.

When choosing whether to start these medications in patients with T2DM and established cardiovascular disease, there are several important considerations. Liraglutide is a once-daily injectable requiring injection teaching and may pose greater challenges to adherence than a daily tablet. Empagliflozin, prescribed in 10-mg and 25-mg once-daily tablets, may be an attractive alternative, although it is not known if the 10-mg dose would be similarly effective in an adequately powered trial.

The adverse effects and contraindications of liraglutide and empagliflozin also should be considered. Liraglutide can have gastrointestinal side effects, such as nausea, vomiting, and diarrhea, that may make it poorly tolerated by patients already on medications (like metformin), which can cause similar side effects. Liraglutide also may increase the risk for acute pancreatitis, and it cannot be given to patients with medullary thyroid cancer or with personal or family history of MEN type 2.

Empagliflozin carries increased risk for dehydration and genital infections, and thus health care providers should stress the importance of drinking water and maintaining good hygiene with patients taking this medication. Empagliflozin should not be given to patients with severe renal impairment, end-stage renal disease, or in dialysis patients, and the FDA recommends discontinuing the drug if eGFR falls to below 45 mL/min per 1.73 m^2 due to increased risk of adverse events with impaired renal function. Importantly, clinicians also should be mindful of the potential for patients on either liraglutide or empagliflozin to develop hypoglycemia, as both these medications reduce blood glucose levels, and the risk for hypoglycemia is increased when given with other antidiabetes medications.

These new agents bring promise for patients with T2DM at risk for cardiovascular events, and require we have discussions on how best to manage these patients. Should cardiologists learn how to treat patients with T2DM? Alternatively, should we develop multispecialty clinics, in which there is subspecialty expertise from cardiology, endocrinology, and nephrology to best manage this large population? At minimum, communication among these subspecialties will have to be streamlined. These ideas suggest a major paradigm shift in the management of cardiovascular disease and diabetes, an undertaking that poses many logistical questions.

Last, it is not clear the role that aggressive lifestyle change had in this group, as the degree and success of lifestyle change was not reported in either study. Lifestyle changes are important but often overlooked interventions both in development and prevention of cardiovascular disease, and warrant further investigation.

REFERENCES

1. Tancredi M, Rosengren A, Svensson AM, et al. Excess mortality among persons with type 2 diabetes. N Engl J Med 2015;373(18):1720–32.
2. Das SR, Everett BM, Birtcher KK, et al. ACC Expert consensus decision pathway on novel therapies for cardiovascular risk reduction in patients with type 2 diabetes and atherosclerotic cardiovascular disease. Am J Cardiol 2018;72(24):3200–23.
3. Garber AJ, Abrahamson MJ, Barzilay JI, et al. Consensus statement by the American Association of Clinical Endocrinologists and American College of Endocrinology on the comprehensive type 2 diabetes management algorithm - 2018 executive summary. Endocr Pract 2018;24:91–120.
4. Cavero-Redondo I, Peleteiro B, Álvarez-Bueno C, et al. Glycated haemoglobin A1c as a risk factor of cardiovascular outcomes and all-cause mortality in diabetic and non-diabetic populations: a systematic review and meta-analysis. BMJ Open 2017;7(7). https://doi.org/10.1136/bmjopen-2017-015949.
5. Udell JA, Farkouh ME, Richard S. Glucose-lowering drugs or strategies and cardiovascular outcomes in patients with or at risk for type 2 diabetes: a meta-analysis of randomised controlled trials. Lancet Diabetes Endocrinol 2015;3:356–66.
6. U.S. Food and Drug Administration. Guidance for industry diabetes mellitus—evaluating cardiovascular risk in new antidiabetic therapies to treat type 2 diabetes. Available at: http://www.fda.gov/cder/guidance/index.htm. Accessed November 11, 2018.
7. Zinman B, Wanner C, Lachin JM, et al. Empagliflozin, cardiovascular outcomes, and mortality in type 2 diabetes. N Engl J Med 2015;373(22):2117–28.
8. Marso SP, Daniels GH, Brown-Frandsen K, et al. Liraglutide and cardiovascular outcomes in type 2 diabetes. N Engl J Med 2016;374:311–22.
9. Marso SP, Poulter NR, Nissen SE, et al. Design of the liraglutide effect and action in diabetes: evaluation of cardiovascular outcome results (LEADER) trial. Am Heart J 2013;166(5):823–30.

10. Zinman B, Inzucchi SE, Lachin JM, et al. Rationale, design, and baseline characteristics of a randomized, placebo-controlled cardiovascular outcome trial of empagliflozin (EMPA-REG OUTCOME™). Cardiovasc Diabetol 2014;13(1):102.

11. Garg SK, Henry RR, Banks P, et al. Effects of sotagliflozin added to insulin in patients with type 1 diabetes. N Engl J Med 2017;377(24): 2337–48.

12. Zelniker TA, Braunwald E. Cardiac and renal effects of sodium-glucose co-transporter 2 inhibitors in diabetes. J Am Coll Cardiol 2018;72(15): 1845–55.

13. Schumi J, Wittes JT. Through the looking glass: understanding non-inferiority. Trials 2011;12:106.

14. Hey SP, Weijer C. Assay sensitivity and the epistemic contexts of clinical trials. Perspect Biol Med 2013;56(1):1–17.

15. Fitchett D, Inzucchi SE, Lachin JM, et al, EMPA-REG OUTCOME Investigators. Cardiovascular mortality reduction with empagliflozin in patients with type 2 diabetes and cardiovascular disease. Am J Cardiol 2018;71(3):364–7.

16. Wanner C, Inzucchi SE, Lachin JM, et al. Empagliflozin and progression of kidney disease in type 2 diabetes. N Engl J Med 2016;375(4):323–34.

17. Wanner C, Lachin JM, Inzucchi SE, et al, EMPA-REG OUTCOME Investigators. Empagliflozin and clinical outcomes in patients with type 2 diabetes mellitus, established cardiovascular disease, and chronic kidney disease. Circulation 2018;137(2): 119–29.

18. Lee YS, Jun HS. Anti-diabetic actions of glucagon-like peptide-1 on pancreatic beta-cells. Metabolism 2014;63(1):9–19.

19. Mann JFE, Fonseca V, Mosenzon O, et al. Effects of liraglutide versus placebo on cardiovascular events in patients with type 2 diabetes and chronic kidney disease: results from the LEADER trial. Circulation 2018;138(25):2908–18.

20. Worcester S, Otto MA, Nogrady B. FDA advisory committee supports new CV liraglutide indication. MDedge Psychiatry. 2018. Available at: https://www.mdedge.com/cardiology/article/140962/diabetes/fda-advisory-committee-supports-new-cv-liraglutide-indication. Accessed December 21, 2018.

21. Rutten GE, Tack CJ, Pieber TR, et al. LEADER 7: cardiovascular risk profiles of US and European participants in the LEADER diabetes trial differ. Diabetol Metab Syndr 2016;8:37.

FURTHER READINGS

Jardiance Highlights of Prescribing Information.n.d. Available at: https://docs.boehringer-ingelheim.com/Prescribing%20Information/PIs/Jardiance/jardiance.pdf.

Saxenda (liraglutide [rDNA origin] injection) Prescribing Information.n.d. Available at: https://www.accessdata.fda.gov/drugsatfda_docs/label/2014/206321Orig1s000lbl.pdf.

Victoza (liraglutide) Full Prescribing Information.n.d. Available at: https://www.novo-pi.com/victoza.pdf.

Hypertensive Disorders of Pregnancy

Silvi Shah, MD, MS[a],*, Anu Gupta, MD[b]

KEYWORDS

- Hypertension • Pregnancy • Preeclampsia • Treatment

KEY POINTS

- Hypertensive disorders of pregnancy complicate up to 15% of pregnancies and remain the leading cause of maternal mortality.
- Preeclampsia is a pregnancy-specific hypertensive disorder with multisystem involvement and is associated with future cardiovascular disease risk.
- Management of preeclampsia involves early recognition and timely delivery.
- Treatment of hypertension during pregnancy is recommended when systolic pressure is greater than or equal to 150 mm Hg or diastolic pressure is greater than or equal to 100 mm Hg.
- Labetalol, nifedipine, or methyldopa is the recommended first-line antihypertensive drug in pregnant women.

INTRODUCTION

Hypertension is the most commonly observed medical disorder seen during pregnancy and complicates up to 15% of pregnancies in women of childbearing age.[1,2] Worldwide, hypertensive disorders remain the leading causes of pregnancy-related maternal mortality.[3,4] In the United States, hypertensive disorders contribute to 7% to 12% pregnancy-related maternal deaths.[4,5] Hypertensive disorders of pregnancy are classified into 4 categories, as recommended by the National High Blood Pressure Education Program Working Group Report on High Blood Pressure in Pregnancy and the American College of Obstetrics and Gynecology (ACOG): (1) chronic hypertension, (2) preeclampsia, (3) preeclampsia superimposed on chronic hypertension, and (4) gestational hypertension.[1,2] White coat hypertension is included as an additional category by some societies like the International Society for the Study of Hypertension in Pregnancy in their guidelines.[6] Women with

hypertensive disorders of pregnancy have a 2-times higher risk of developing cardiovascular disease than those who are normotensive during pregnancy.[7] Under the physiologic stress test of pregnancy, hypertensive disorders of pregnancy may provide early insight into cardiovascular risk and help identify high-risk women for targeted prevention.[8] Hypertensive disorders of pregnancy also are associated with impaired glucose tolerance and insulin resistance and a 3-fold to 4-fold increased risk for diabetes mellitus type 2.[9,10] History of nephrolithiasis is associated with higher risk of hypertensive disorders of pregnancy, especially in women with high first-trimester body mass index.[11] Because hypertensive disorders of pregnancy increase the risk of maternal and perinatal mortality and morbidity, timely diagnosis and proper treatment are essential to preventing these complications.[12,13] In this review, the authors describe the most recent updates on the classification of hypertensive disorders of pregnancy, latest findings on pathogenesis and implications of

Disclosure Statement: The authors have nothing to disclose.
[a] Division of Nephrology, Kidney CARE Program, University of Cincinnati, 231 Albert Sabin Way, MSB 6211, Cincinnati, OH 45267, USA; [b] Buffalo Medical Group, 2121 Main Street #305, Buffalo, NY 14214, USA
* Corresponding author.
E-mail address: shah2sv@ucmail.uc.edu

preeclampsia, and summary of treatment strategies of hypertension during pregnancy.

CHRONIC HYPERTENSION

Chronic hypertension complicates approximately 3% to 5% of pregnancies in United States, and the prevalence rates are increasing over time, with primary drivers an increase in obesity and delay in childbearing age.[14] Chronic hypertension is defined by systolic blood pressure greater than or equal to 140 mm Hg and/or diastolic blood pressure of greater than or equal to 90 mm Hg present before pregnancy or on at least 2 occasions before 20 weeks of gestation.[15] Importantly, secondary causes in women diagnosed with chronic hypertension should be ruled out. Women may experience a physiologic lowering of blood pressure during pregnancy due to the systemic vasodilation and a reduction in the requirement for antihypertensive medications. This nadir in blood pressure, especially in the second trimester, can result in diagnostic uncertainty.[16]

Although blood pressure may return to normal during the postpartum period, hypertension during pregnancy is associated with risk of future chronic hypertension.[17] Approximately 25% of women with chronic hypertension develop preeclampsia during pregnancy.[18] Due to additional risk with superimposed preeclampsia, chronic hypertension accounts for significant maternal and perinatal morbidity and mortality. Compared with the general population, women with chronic hypertension have higher rates of caesarean sections (41%), preterm births (28%), low birth weights (17%), neonatal intensive care unit admissions (21%), and perinatal mortality (4.0%).[12] These women, therefore, should undergo increased surveillance and serial laboratory tests and ultrasound scans to follow growth during the course of their pregnancies.[14]

PREECLAMPSIA
Diagnosis

Preeclampsia is a pregnancy-specific hypertensive disorder with multisystem involvement. Preeclampsia affects approximately 2% to 8% of pregnancies worldwide. In the United States, the rate of preeclampsia is approximately 3.4%.[19] Diagnosis is made by new onset of hypertension after 20 weeks of gestation in a previously normotensive woman defined by blood pressure greater than or equal to 140/90 mm Hg on 2 occasions 4 hours apart, or greater than or equal to 160/110 mm Hg within a shorter interval, and proteinuria greater than or equal to 300-mg/24-hour urine or spot urine

protein:creatinine ratio of 0.3 (dipstick 1+). Preeclampsia can be diagnosed in the absence of proteinuria if any of the following signs of end-organ dysfunction are present: elevated serum creatinine greater than 1.1 mg/dL or doubling of serum creatinine in the absence of other renal disease, thrombocytopenia (<100,000/μL), elevated liver transaminases greater than or equal to 2 times normal, pulmonary edema, or cerebral/visual symptoms.[2,20] The most common presentation of preeclampsia is detection of hypertension at a routine antenatal visit in an asymptomatic woman. Symptoms (visual complaints, headache, vomiting, and abdominal pain) and signs (altered mental status, papilledema, hyperreflexia with marked clonus, pulmonary edema, and right upper quadrant tenderness) are usually seen with severe preeclampsia defined by severe hypertension (blood pressure >160/110 mm Hg) with evidence of end-organ damage.[2,21,22] The risk of adverse outcomes increases significantly when preeclampsia develops early, before 34 weeks' gestation. Due to the highly diverse phenotypic spectrum and some common features, a diagnosis of preeclampsia can be challenging in the setting of preexisting hypertension or kidney disease. It has been suggested, however, that the angiogenic markers, soluble fms-like tyrosine kinase 1 (sFlt-1) and placental growth factor (PlGF), may be able to distinguish preeclampsia from chronic kidney disease.[23]

Risk Factors

Risk factors include maternal age greater than or equal to 40, obesity, diabetes mellitus, chronic hypertension, obesity, chronic kidney disease, systemic lupus erythematous, presence of antiphospholipid antibodies, nulliparity, multiple gestations, high altitude, prior history of preeclampsia, and family history of preeclampsia or cardiovascular disease.[24,25] History of clinically recovered acute kidney injury increases the risk of preeclampsia by 4.7-fold.[26] Tangren and colleagues[11] in a retrospective cohort study showed that preeclampsia was more common in stone formers than non–stone formers (16% vs 8%), and previous nephrolithiasis was associated with 2.2-fold higher risk of preeclampsia. History of living kidney donation increases the risk of preeclampsia by 2.4-fold.[27] Kidney transplant recipients 6-fold higher risk of preeclampsia, and the incidence ranges between 24% and 38%.[28]

Maternal and Fetal Complications

Preeclampsia remains the leading cause of maternal and perinatal mortality and morbidity.[29,30]

Preeclampsia can lead to neurologic complications, such as seizures (eclampsia) and strokes, kidney injury, and the hemolysis, elevated liver enzymes and low platelets (HELLP) syndrome.[31,32] The HELLP syndrome occurs in approximately 10% to 20% of women with severe preeclampsia.[33]

Preeclampsia is a state of physiologic insulin resistance and is independently associated with 2.4-fold higher risk of future diabetes. Wu and colleagues[10] demonstrated in their meta-analysis that the risk of diabetes with preeclampsia persisted in studies that followed women from less than 1 year postpartum (relative risk [RR] 1.97, 95% CI, 1.35–2.87) to more than 10 years postpartum (RR 1.95, 95% CI, 1.28–2.97). The prevalence of the metabolic syndrome in is 2-fold higher for women with a history of preeclampsia.[34] The association between preeclampsia and cardiovascular diseases is well known. Women with history of preeclampsia have a 3.7-times higher risk of developing hypertension, a 2.2-times increased risk of coronary heart disease, and a 1.8-times higher risk of stroke later in life.[35] A study by McDonald and colleagues[7] showed that preeclamptic women have higher risk of cardiac disease (RR 2.33, 95% CI, 1.95 to 2.78), cerebrovascular disease (RR 2.03, 95% CI, 1.54–2.67), peripheral arterial disease (RR 1.87, 95% CI, 0.94–3.73), and cardiovascular mortality (RR 2.29, 95% CI, 1.73–3.04). Peripartum cardiomyopathy can be seen in women with preeclampsia. The pathophysiologic relation between preeclampsia and subsequent cardiovascular disease, although unclear, has been hypothesized to proinflammatory activity, impaired endothelial function, and increased insulin resistance.[36,37]

Additionally, preeclampsia is associated with cumulative risk of subsequent end-stage kidney disease (ESKD). Vikse and colleagues[38] showed that among women who had been pregnant 1 or more times, preeclampsia during the first pregnancy was associated with a 4.7-fold higher risk of ESKD. Preeclampsia during the first pregnancy was associated with 3.2-fold higher risk of ESKD and preeclampsia during the second pregnancy was associated with 6.7-fold higher risk of ESKD in women with 2 or more pregnancies.

Preeclampsia can be complicated by placental abruption oligohydramnios, cesarean delivery, and preterm delivery. Fetal growth restriction is seen in up to 30% of the pregnancies.[39–42] Preeclampsia predisposes the children of affected mothers to exaggerated hypoxic pulmonary hypertension and development of premature cardiovascular disease in the systemic circulation. Jayet and colleagues[43] showed that pulmonary artery pressure was approximately 30% higher in offspring of women with preeclampsia compared with children born to mothers without preeclampsia. Preeclampsia is an important risk factor for bronchopulmonary dysplasia development, possibly due to its antiangiogenic state.[44] The incidence of bronchopulmonary dysplasia was significantly higher in preterm infants born to preeclamptic women than in those born to normotensive women (38.5% vs 19.5%, respectively).[45]

Pathophysiology

Although the pathogenesis of preeclampsia is not fully elucidated, the etiologic processes are affected by maternal, genetic, immunologic, and environmental factors.

Placenta plays a central role in the pathogenesis of preeclampsia, which is believed to be initiated by placental ischemia followed by placental release of antiangiogenic factors into the circulation. During normal pregnancy, to improve the circulation between fetus and mother, the placenta undergoes vascularization that involves vasculogenesis, angiogenesis, and maternal spiral artery remodeling. The cytotrophoblasts invade the maternal spiral arterioles and remodel them into large capacitance vessels with low resistance.[46] The endovascular cytotrophoblast invasion involves replacement of both the endothelium and the highly muscular tunica media. The trophoblasts alter their adhesion molecule expression from epithelial cells to endothelial cells, such as those from the vascular endothelial growth factor (VEGF) family, which is important for uterine invasion, and is referred to as *pseudovasculogenesis*. The formation of this uteroplacental unit increases the supply of oxygen and nutrients to the fetus.[47,48] In preeclampsia, however, pseudovasculogenesis is incomplete due to shallow placental cytotrophoblast invasion of uterine spiral arterioles, thus resulting in impaired placental perfusion and release of hypoxia inducible factors. Furthermore, the expression of VEGF family of molecules is down-regulated, and the expression of its inhibitors is up-regulated.[49]

The molecular pathway that regulates pseudovasculogenesis involves a vast array of transcription factors, growth factors, and cytokines.[50] The normal placenta produces a balance of proangiogenic VEGF and PIGF and antiangiogenic factors (sFlt-1). VEGF, a proangiogenic factor, is expressed by the placenta and binds to its specific receptors on placental cells and on vascular endothelial cells.[51,52] PIGF is produced by trophoblasts and, through binding to sFlt-1 receptor, plays an important role in vasculogenesis and vasodilation.

An imbalance between different proangiogenic and antiangiogenic factors is the inciting event in the onset of preeclampsia. sFlt-1 levels are elevated in the preeclamptic women, and this up-regulation is associated with decreased levels of circulating free VEGF and free PlGF. sFlt1 is a circulating decoy receptor that binds to PlGF and leads to endothelial dysfunction by preventing its interaction with cell surface receptors.[53] Similarly, another antiangiogenic protein, soluble endoglin (sEng), is up-regulated in preeclampsia. sEng binds to the transforming growth factor β and prohibits transforming growth factor β signaling in trophoblasts, which leads to poor placentation. The elevated levels of sEng levels correlate with disease severity in preeclamptic individuals.[54] Relaxin, a peptide hormone, produced by the corpus luteum of the ovary, rises early in pregnancy. Relaxin up-regulates vascular gelatinase activity during gestation, thereby contributing to renal vasodilation, hyperfiltration, and reduced myogenic reactivity of small renal arteries.[55] Low first-trimester relaxin levels have been found in first trimester of pregnancy in patients with preeclampsia.[56]

Additionally, maternal and paternal genes have been postulated as having a role in defective placentation. The incidence of preeclampsia is significantly higher in trisomy 13 pregnancies than in normal pregnancies. Elevated sFlt-1 and reduced PlGF have been found with trisomy 13 pregnancies.[57] Although preeclampsia seems to originate in placenta, the tissue most affected is the maternal endothelium. The clinical manifestations of preeclampsia reflect widespread endothelial dysfunction with vasoconstriction and end-organ ischemia. The hallmark renal pathology in preeclampsia is glomerular endotheliosis.[58]

Diagnostic Markers

Preeclampsia is associated with an abnormal pattern of circulating maternal proangiogenic and antiangiogenic factors that disrupt the proper angiogenic balance (PlGF, sEng, and sFlt-1). Recent research has been targeted to identify angiogenic factors as either predictive or diagnostic biomarkers of preeclampsia. Increase in serum sFlt-1 levels and decrease in PlGF level occur in preeclamptic women many weeks preceding the manifestation of the disease. Levine and colleagues[53] performed a nested case-control study in 120 pairs of women, where each woman with preeclampsia was matched to 1 normotensive control. The study showed a mean sFlt-1 value of 4382 pg/mL versus 1643 pg/mL and a mean serum PlGF concentration of 137 pg/mL versus 669 pg/mL at the disease onset in preeclamptic women as compared to healthy control pregnancies. In the Calcium for Preeclampsia Prevention trial, the mean sEng levels of women with preterm and term preeclampsia were found significantly higher than in healthy control pregnancies.[59] Zeisler and colleagues[60] demonstrated that sFlt-1:PlGF ratio cutoff of 38 had a negative predictive value of 99.3%, sensitivity of 80%, and specificity of 78.3% and can be used to predict the short-term absence of preeclampsia in women with clinical suspicion. This approach needs to be validated in prospective studies with larger numbers of patients, and a screening test for preeclampsia is still not available.[61,62]

Prevention

Because delivery is the only curative treatment of preeclampsia, early identification followed by appropriate management may prevent life-threatening complications of preeclampsia. Screening for hypertension should be performed at every prenatal visit.[63] Low-dose aspirin reduces the risk of preeclampsia by 10% to 20% and lowers the risk of adverse pregnancy outcomes of preterm birth and growth restriction. Prophylaxis with aspirin should be started at greater than or equal to 12 weeks of gestation and ideally prior to 16 weeks in women at high risk of developing preeclampsia.[64] Roberge and colleagues[65] performed a meta-analysis that included 45 randomized controlled trials and 20,909 pregnant women. Aspirin initiated at less than or equal to 16 weeks was associated with reduction in the risk of preeclampsia in a dose-response effect (RR 0.57; 95% CI, 0.43–0.75), severe preeclampsia (RR 0.47; 95% CI, 0.26–0.83), and fetal growth restriction (RR 0.56; 95% CI, 0.44–0.70). The higher dosages of aspirin were associated with greater reduction of the 3 outcomes and low-dose aspirin initiated at greater than 16 weeks' gestation has a moderate or no impact on the risk of preeclampsia. Pregnant women should achieve the recommended daily calcium allowance of 1000 mg daily to reduce the risk of preeclampsia. In populations with baseline low calcium intake, it is recommended to give 1500 mg to 2000 mg elemental calcium supplementation per day for pregnant women to reduce the risk of preeclampsia.[66,67] Use of folic acid in reducing the risk of preeclampsia is unclear, however folic is given prior to conception to prevent neural tube defects.[68]

PREECLAMPSIA SUPERIMPOSED ON CHRONIC HYPERTENSION

Superimposed preeclampsia is diagnosed in women with a prior history of hypertension who demonstrate worsening of hypertension and development of new-onset proteinuria after 20 weeks' gestation. A rise in blood pressure and the need for antihypertensive therapy in the third trimester are not unexpected in women with preexisting essential hypertension; hence, hypertension alone is not sufficient to diagnose preeclampsia, and only if a woman develops worsening hypertension in combination with proteinuria, new organ dysfunction, or uteroplacental dysfunction may preeclampsia then be diagnosed confidently. A diagnosis of preeclampsia remains most challenging in women with long-standing hypertension and renal impairment. Because approximately 25% of pregnancies in women with chronic hypertension are complicated by superimposed preeclampsia, close monitoring is recommended.[69]

GESTATIONAL HYPERTENSION

Gestational hypertension is the most common cause of hypertension during pregnancy and is defined by the onset of hypertension (systolic blood pressure $\geq$140 mm Hg and/or diastolic blood pressure $\geq$90 mm Hg) after 20 weeks of gestation without proteinuria or absence of new signs of end-organ dysfunction. The diagnosis is modified to preeclampsia with new onset of proteinuria or end-organ dysfunction and to chronic hypertension when elevation in blood pressure elevation persists greater than or equal to 12 weeks postpartum.[2,40] History of preeclampsia, multiple gestation, and obesity are some of the important risk factors associated with the onset of gestational hypertension. Approximately 10% to 50% of women with gestational hypertension develop preeclampsia during the course of pregnancy.[70] Severe gestational hypertension also is associated with higher rates of preterm delivery and delivery of small-for-gestational-age infants than women.[71] Gestational age less than 34 weeks, mean systolic blood pressure greater than 135 mm Hg, abnormal uterine artery Doppler velocimetry, and elevated serum uric acid level (>5.2 mg/dL) increase the risk of progression to preeclampsia.[70] Women with gestational hypertension should undergo increased surveillance during pregnancy, and reassessment at 12 weeks postpartum should be done to establish the final diagnosis.[2] **Table 1** shows the diagnostic features of different subtypes of hypertensive disorders of pregnancy.

TREATMENT

The thresholds of starting treatment, targets, and choice of antihypertensive medications are different in pregnant women compared with nonpregnant individuals. Treatment of severe hypertension reduces the risk of maternal stroke, but the maternal and fetal benefits from treatment of mild to moderate hypertension during the short duration of a full-term pregnancy remain unclear. Lowering of maternal blood pressure excessively may be associated with reduced placental perfusion. Additionally, use of antihypertensive medication may have potential adverse effects to the fetus.[72] In a Cochrane meta-analysis done by Abalos and colleagues,[72] including 31 trials and 3485 pregnant women with mild to moderate hypertension (defined as systolic blood pressure 140–169 mm Hg and/or diastolic 90–109 mm Hg), it was found that the use of antihypertensive medications reduced the risk of severe hypertension by almost half but had little or no effect on the risk of proteinuria and preeclampsia. Magee and colleagues[73] conducted a multicenter trial (Control of Hypertension in Pregnancy Study [CHIPS]) and 987 women with chronic or gestational hypertension were randomly assigned to less tight control (target diastolic blood pressure, 100 mm Hg) or tight control (target diastolic blood pressure, 85 mm Hg). The study showed no significant differences in the risk of pregnancy loss, high-level neonatal care, or overall maternal complications between the 2 groups. Less tight control was associated, however, with a significantly higher frequency of severe maternal hypertension. In a post hoc analysis of the CHIPS trial, severe maternal hypertension was associated with lower infant birth weight and with more preterm delivery, preeclampsia, and features of HELLP syndrome.[74] Treatment-induced falls in maternal blood pressure may affect fetal growth adversely. In a meta-analysis done by von Dadelszen and colleagues,[75] greater treatment-induced mean difference in maternal mean arterial pressure was found associated with a higher proportion of small for gestational age infants.

The guidelines for the management of hypertension in pregnancy differ with respect to threshold for initiation of treatment. The ACOG suggests treatment of persistent chronic hypertension when systolic pressure is greater than or equal to 160 mm Hg or diastolic pressure is greater than or equal to 110 mm Hg.[2] According to the Canadian Hypertensive Disorders of Pregnancy Working Group, therapy is recommended in pregnant women with no comorbid conditions, targeting systolic blood pressure at 130 mm Hg to 155 mm Hg and diastolic pressure at 80 mm Hg to 105 mm Hg.[76] Based on the results of the CHIPS trial, the authors agree with initiating antihypertensive therapy in adult women with chronic

Table 1
Classification of hypertensive disorders of pregnancy

	Time of Diagnosis	Diagnostic Features
Chronic hypertension	<20 wk	Hypertension ($\geq$140/90 mm Hg) present prior to conception or diagnosed <20 wk
Gestational hypertension	>20 wk	New-onset hypertension with absence of proteinuria
Preeclampsia	>20 wk	New-onset hypertension and proteinuria ($\geq$300 mg/24 h) or new-onset hypertension with end-organ dysfunction in the absence of proteinuria
Preeclampsia superimposed on chronic hypertension	>20 wk	Worsening hypertension with new onset of proteinuria or features of end-organ dysfunction

hypertension at systolic pressures greater than or equal to 150 mm Hg or diastolic blood pressures greater than or equal to 100 mm Hg and maintaining systolic blood pressure at 130 mm Hg to 150 mm Hg and diastolic blood pressure at and 80 mm Hg to 100 mm Hg. In women with target organ damage, keeping the blood pressure below 140/90 mm Hg should be considered.[15] For women with chronic hypertension and mild to moderately increased blood pressures before pregnancy, it is reasonable to expect that pressures may decrease early in pregnancy, owing to physiologic vasodilation, and, if there is no known target organ damage, clinicians can consider discontinuing or tapering antihypertensive treatment and monitoring, provided patients are followed-up closely.[77]

In preeclampsia, both the gestational age and the level of blood pressure influence the use of antihypertensive therapy. Management of preeclampsia includes early recognition and timely delivery.[20] Although the primary underlying pathophysiologic process is not reversed with blood pressure control, severe hypertension in pregnancy, defined as greater than 160/110 mm Hg, always should be treated to prevent the maternal complications of intracerebral hemorrhage and maternal death.[78] Therapy should be individualized based on maternal and fetal factors, and targets include systolic blood pressure between 130 mm Hg and 150 mm Hg and diastolic blood pressure between 80 mm Hg and 100 mm Hg.[79] Acute-onset severe hypertension associated with eclampsia, hemorrhage, or hypertensive encephalopathy requires emergent therapy with parenteral agents, with a goal of lowering mean arterial pressure by 25% within minutes to hours. Caution should be given to the rapidity with which blood pressure is lowered. Fetal distress and cerebral or myocardial ischemia can occur if the blood pressure falls below the range at which tissue perfusion and placental blood flow is autoregulated. Initiating treatment in acute severe hypertension at lower doses should be considered, because patients with severe hypertension during pregnancy are intravascularly volume depleted and may be at increased risk for hypotension.[80]

First-line antihypertensive in pregnant women includes labetalol, nifedipine, and methyldopa. Methyldopa has been used extensively in pregnant women and its long-term safety has been documented.[81] Methyldopa has slow onset of action, within 3 hours to 6 hours, and acts via central α_2 blocking effect. Side effects include decreased mental alertness and salivation, xerostomia, and elevated liver enzymes. Labetalol is a β-blocker with both α-adrenergic and β-adrenergic blocking activity and may preserve uteroplacental blood flow to a greater extent compared with traditional β-blockers.[82] Atenolol is contraindicated for use in pregnancy due to its association with intrauterine growth restriction.[83] Long-acting nifedipine has been shown safe for use in chronic hypertension in pregnancy but is associated with side effects of palpitations, peripheral edema, headaches, and facial flushing.[84] Renin angiotensin system inhibitors and direct renin inhibitors are contraindicated during pregnancy due to the risk of fetal renal abnormalities and cardiovascular and central nervous system malformation associated with its exposure.[85] Spironolactone is not recommended for use during pregnancy, because of its antiandrogenic effects during fetal development.[86] The role of thiazide diuretics in pregnancy is controversial. Thiazide diuretics may be continued through pregnancy in women who had

Table 2
Pharmacologic therapy for hypertensive disorders in pregnancy

		Risks
Central agents		
Preferred	Methyldopa	Neurodepressant side effects, decreased mental alertness, dry mouth, xerostomia, elevated liver enzymes, potentiates postpartum depression
Alternative	Clonidine	Unproved safety
β-Blockers		
Preferred	Labetalol	Fetal bradycardia, neonatal hypoglycemia
Contraindicated	Atenolol	Intrauterine growth retardation
Calcium channel blockers		
Preferred	Nifedipine	Headache, tachycardia, palpitations, facial flushing, peripheral edema, profound hypotension with magnesium
Alternative	Verapamil	Unproved safety profile
Direct vasodilators		
Preferred	Hydralazine	Headache, flushing, maternal neuropathy, drug-induced lupus syndrome
Alternative	Nitroprusside	Cyanide toxicity
Diuretics		
Preferred	Thiazides	Volume contraction
Contraindicated	Spironolactone	Fetal antiandrogen affect and ambiguous genitalia
Renin angiotensinogen system inhibitors		
Contraindicated	Angiotensin-converting enzyme inhibitors and angiotensin II receptor blocker antagonists	Renal dysgenesis, oligohydramnios, pulmonary hypoplasia, cardiovascular and central nervous system malformation

been taking them prior to conception. Diuretics affect the plasma volume expansion of normal pregnancy but have not been associated with a negative effect on fetal growth.[87] First-line medications for acute therapy for severe hypertension in pregnancy include intravenous labetalol and hydralazine.

Adverse effects include headache, flushing, and palpitations due to vasodilation or sympathetic activation.[88] Nitroprusside is used as a last resort for control of refractory severe hypertension due to the risk of cyanide toxicity. Caution should be exercised with the use of immediate-release oral nifedipine because it can cause acute drop of blood pressure and hypotension.[80,81] **Table 2** elucidates the safety profile of the various antihypertensive drugs for use in pregnancy.

This review summarizes the pathophysiology, diagnosis, and management of hypertensive disorders of pregnancy. Preeclampsia is associated with high risk of maternal mortality and its management requires a multidisciplinary approach between nephrologists, high-risk maternal fetal medicine obstetrician, and neonatologist. Women who develop hypertensive complications in pregnancy should be followed closely postpartum and counseled for increased risk of future cardiovascular disease.

REFERENCES

1. National High Blood Pressure Education Program. Report of the national high blood pressure education program working group on high blood pressure in pregnancy. Am J Obstet Gynecol 2000; 183:s1–22.

2. Hypertension in pregnancy. Report of the American College of obstetricians and Gynecologists' task force on hypertension in pregnancy. Obstet Gynecol 2013;122:1122–31.

3. Leffert LR, Clancy CR, Bateman BT, et al. Hypertensive disorders and pregnancy-related stroke: frequency, trends, risk factors, and outcomes. Obstet Gynecol 2015;125:124–31.

4. Berg CJ, Callaghan WM, Syverson C, et al. Pregnancy-related mortality in the United States, 1998 to 2005. Obstet Gynecol 2010;116:1302–9.

5. Creanga AA, Syverson C, Seed K, et al. Pregnancy-related mortality in the United States, 2011-2013. Obstet Gynecol 2017;130:366–73.

6. Tranquilli AL, Dekker G, Magee L, et al. The classification, diagnosis and management of the hypertensive disorders of pregnancy: a revised statement from the ISSHP. Pregnancy Hypertens 2014;4:97–104.

7. McDonald SD, Malinowski A, Zhou Q, et al. Cardiovascular sequelae of preeclampsia/eclampsia: a systematic review and meta-analyses. Am Heart J 2008;156:918–30.

8. Sattar N, Greer IA. Pregnancy complications and maternal cardiovascular risk: opportunities for intervention and screening? BMJ 2002;325:157–60.

9. Lykke JA, Langhoff-Roos J, Sibai BM, et al. Hypertensive pregnancy disorders and subsequent cardiovascular morbidity and type 2 diabetes mellitus in the mother. Hypertension 2009;53:944–51.

10. Wu P, Kwok CS, Haththotuwa R, et al. Pre-eclampsia is associated with a twofold increase in diabetes: a systematic review and meta-analysis. Diabetologia 2016;59:2518–26.

11. Tangren JS, Powe CE, Ecker J, et al. Metabolic and hypertensive complications of pregnancy in women with nephrolithiasis. Clin J Am Soc Nephrol 2018;13:612–9.

12. Bramham K, Parnell B, Nelson-Piercy C, et al. Chronic hypertension and pregnancy outcomes: systematic review and meta-analysis. BMJ 2014;348:g2301.

13. Chappell LC, Enye S, Seed P, et al. Adverse perinatal outcomes and risk factors for preeclampsia in women with chronic hypertension: a prospective study. Hypertension 2008;51:1002–9.

14. Mammaro A, Carrara S, Cavaliere A, et al. Hypertensive disorders of pregnancy. J Prenatal Med 2009;3:1–5.

15. Sibai BM. Chronic hypertension in pregnancy. Obstet Gynecol 2002;100:369–77.

16. Folk DM. Hypertensive disorders of pregnancy: overview and current recommendations. J Midwifery Womens Health 2018;63:289–300.

17. Mannisto T, Mendola P, Vaarasmaki M, et al. Elevated blood pressure in pregnancy and subsequent chronic disease risk. Circulation 2013;127:681–90.

18. Seely EW, Ecker J. Clinical practice. Chronic hypertension in pregnancy. N Engl J Med 2011;365:439–46.

19. Ananth CV, Keyes KM, Wapner RJ. Pre-eclampsia rates in the United States, 1980-2010: age-period-cohort analysis. BMJ 2013;347:f6564.

20. Mustafa R, Ahmed S, Gupta A, et al. A comprehensive review of hypertension in pregnancy. J Pregnancy 2012;2012:105918.

21. Townsend R, O'Brien P, Khalil A. Current best practice in the management of hypertensive disorders in pregnancy. Integr Blood Press Control 2016;9:79–94.

22. Magee LA, Pels A, Helewa M, et al. Diagnosis, evaluation, and management of the hypertensive disorders of pregnancy: executive summary. J Obstet Gynaecol Can 2014;36:575–6.

23. Rolfo A, Attini R, Nuzzo AM, et al. Chronic kidney disease may be differentially diagnosed from preeclampsia by serum biomarkers. Kidney Int 2013;83:177–81.

24. Duckitt K, Harrington D. Risk factors for preeclampsia at antenatal booking: systematic review of controlled studies. BMJ 2005;330:565.

25. Uzan J, Carbonnel M, Piconne O, et al. Preeclampsia: pathophysiology, diagnosis, and management. Vasc Health Risk Manag 2011;7:467–74.

26. Tangren JS, Powe CE, Ankers E, et al. Pregnancy outcomes after clinical recovery from AKI. J Am Soc Nephrol 2017;28:1566–74.

27. Garg AX, Nevis IF, McArthur E, et al. Gestational hypertension and preeclampsia in living kidney donors. N Engl J Med 2015;372:124–33.

28. Shah S, Verma P. Overview of pregnancy in renal transplant patients. Int J Nephrol 2016;2016:4539342.

29. Duley L. Maternal mortality associated with hypertensive disorders of pregnancy in Africa, Asia, Latin America and the Caribbean. Br J Obstet Gynaecol 1992;99:547–53.

30. Khan KS, Wojdyla D, Say L, et al. WHO analysis of causes of maternal death: a systematic review. Lancet 2006;367:1066–74.

31. Heard AR, Dekker GA, Chan A, et al. Hypertension during pregnancy in South Australia, part 1: pregnancy outcomes. Aust N Z J Obstet Gynaecol 2004;44:404–9.

32. Sibai BM, Mercer B, Sarinoglu C. Severe preeclampsia in the second trimester: recurrence risk and long-term prognosis. Am J Obstet Gynecol 1991;165:1408–12.

33. Sibai BM. Diagnosis, controversies, and management of the syndrome of hemolysis, elevated liver enzymes, and low platelet count. Obstet Gynecol 2004;103:981–91.

34. Al-Nasiry S, Ghossein-Doha C, Polman SE, et al. Metabolic syndrome after pregnancies complicated by pre-eclampsia or small-for-gestational-age: a retrospective cohort. BJOG 2015;122:1818–23.

35. Bellamy L, Casas JP, Hingorani AD, et al. Pre-eclampsia and risk of cardiovascular disease and cancer in later life: systematic review and meta-analysis. BMJ 2007;335:974.

36. Agatisa PK, Ness RB, Roberts JM, et al. Impairment of endothelial function in women with a history of preeclampsia: an indicator of cardiovascular risk.

Am J Physiol Heart Circ Physiol 2004;286: H1389–93.

37. Kaaja RJ, Poyhonen-Alho MK. Insulin resistance and sympathetic overactivity in women. J Hypertens 2006;24:131–41.

38. Vikse BE, Irgens LM, Leivestad T, et al. Preeclampsia and the risk of end-stage renal disease. N Engl J Med 2008;359:800–9.

39. Backes CH, Markham K, Moorehead P, et al. Maternal preeclampsia and neonatal outcomes. J Pregnancy 2011;2011:214365.

40. Hauth JC, Ewell MG, Levine RJ, et al. Pregnancy outcomes in healthy nulliparas who developed hypertension. Calcium for Preeclampsia Prevention Study Group. Obstet Gynecol 2000;95:24–8.

41. Davis EF, Lazdam M, Lewandowski AJ, et al. Cardiovascular risk factors in children and young adults born to preeclamptic pregnancies: a systematic review. Pediatrics 2012;129:e1552–61.

42. Kajantie E, Eriksson JG, Osmond C, et al. Preeclampsia is associated with increased risk of stroke in the adult offspring: the Helsinki birth cohort study. Stroke 2009;40:1176–80.

43. Jayet PY, Rimoldi SF, Stuber T, et al. Pulmonary and systemic vascular dysfunction in young offspring of mothers with preeclampsia. Circulation 2010;122: 488–94.

44. Dravet-Gounot P, Torchin H, Goffinet F, et al. Bronchopulmonary dysplasia in neonates born to mothers with preeclampsia: impact of small for gestational age. PLoS One 2018;13:e0204498.

45. Ozkan H, Cetinkaya M, Koksal N. Increased incidence of bronchopulmonary dysplasia in preterm infants exposed to preeclampsia. J Matern Fetal Neonatal Med 2012;25:2681–5.

46. Gerretsen G, Huisjes HJ, Elema JD. Morphological changes of the spiral arteries in the placental bed in relation to pre-eclampsia and fetal growth retardation. Br J Obstet Gynaecol 1981;88: 876–81.

47. Zhou Y, Damsky CH, Chiu K, et al. Preeclampsia is associated with abnormal expression of adhesion molecules by invasive cytotrophoblasts. J Clin Invest 1993;91:950–60.

48. Zhou Y, Fisher SJ, Janatpour M, et al. Human cytotrophoblasts adopt a vascular phenotype as they differentiate. A strategy for successful endovascular invasion? J Clin Invest 1997;99:2139–51.

49. Zhou Y, McMaster M, Woo K, et al. Vascular endothelial growth factor ligands and receptors that regulate human cytotrophoblast survival are dysregulated in severe preeclampsia and hemolysis, elevated liver enzymes, and low platelets syndrome. Am J Pathol 2002;160:1405–23.

50. Zhou Y, Genbacev O, Fisher SJ. The human placenta remodels the uterus by using a combination of molecules that govern vasculogenesis or

leukocyte extravasation. Ann N Y Acad Sci 2003; 995:73–83.

51. Melincovici CS, Bosca AB, Susman S, et al. Vascular endothelial growth factor (VEGF) - key factor in normal and pathological angiogenesis. Rom J Morphol Embryol 2018;59:455–67.

52. Moghaddas Sani H, Zununi Vahed S, Ardalan M. Preeclampsia: a close look at renal dysfunction. Biomed Pharmacother 2019;109:408–16.

53. Levine RJ, Maynard SE, Qian C, et al. Circulating angiogenic factors and the risk of preeclampsia. N Engl J Med 2004;350:672–83.

54. Venkatesha S, Toporsian M, Lam C, et al. Soluble endoglin contributes to the pathogenesis of preeclampsia. Nat Med 2006;12:642–9.

55. Jeyabalan A, Novak J, Danielson LA, et al. Essential role for vascular gelatinase activity in relaxin-induced renal vasodilation, hyperfiltration, and reduced myogenic reactivity of small arteries. Circ Res 2003;93:1249–57.

56. Conrad KP. Emerging role of relaxin in the maternal adaptations to normal pregnancy: implications for preeclampsia. Semin Nephrol 2011;31:15–32.

57. Kakigano A, Mimura K, Kanagawa T, et al. Imbalance of angiogenic factors and avascular edematous cystic villi in a trisomy 13 pregnancy: a case report. Placenta 2013;34:628–30.

58. Stillman IE, Karumanchi SA. The glomerular injury of preeclampsia. J Am Soc Nephrol 2007;18:2281–4.

59. Levine RJ, Lam C, Qian C, et al. Soluble endoglin and other circulating antiangiogenic factors in preeclampsia. N Engl J Med 2006;355: 992–1005.

60. Zeisler H, Llurba E, Chantraine F, et al. Predictive value of the sFlt-1:PlGF ratio in women with suspected preeclampsia. N Engl J Med 2016;374: 13–22.

61. Romero R, Nien JK, Espinoza J, et al. A longitudinal study of angiogenic (placental growth factor) and anti-angiogenic (soluble endoglin and soluble vascular endothelial growth factor receptor-1) factors in normal pregnancy and patients destined to develop preeclampsia and deliver a small for gestational age neonate. J Matern Fetal Neonatal Med 2008;21:9–23.

62. Verlohren S, Galindo A, Schlembach D, et al. An automated method for the determination of the sFlt-1/PlGF ratio in the assessment of preeclampsia. Am J Obstet Gynecol 2010;202:161.e1-11.

63. Sperling JD, Gossett DR. Screening for preeclampsia and the USPSTF recommendations. JAMA 2017;317:1629–30.

64. Meher S, Duley L, Hunter K, et al. Antiplatelet therapy before or after 16 weeks' gestation for preventing preeclampsia: an individual participant data meta-analysis. Am J Obstet Gynecol 2017;216: 121–8.e2.

65. Roberge S, Nicolaides K, Demers S, et al. The role of aspirin dose on the prevention of preeclampsia and fetal growth restriction: systematic review and meta-analysis. Am J Obstet Gynecol 2017;216:110–20.e6.

66. Hofmeyr GJ, Lawrie TA, Atallah AN, et al. Calcium supplementation during pregnancy for preventing hypertensive disorders and related problems. Cochrane Database Syst Rev 2014;(6):CD001059.

67. Hofmeyr GJ, Lawrie TA, Atallah AN, et al. Calcium supplementation during pregnancy for preventing hypertensive disorders and related problems. Cochrane Database Syst Rev 2018;(10):CD001059.

68. Hua X, Zhang J, Guo Y, et al. Effect of folic acid supplementation during pregnancy on gestational hypertension/preeclampsia: a systematic review and meta-analysis. Hypertens Pregnancy 2016;35: 447–60.

69. Ankumah NE, Sibai BM. Chronic hypertension in pregnancy: diagnosis, management, and outcomes. Clin Obstet Gynecol 2017;60:206–14.

70. Melamed N, Ray JG, Hladunewich M, et al. Gestational hypertension and preeclampsia: are they the same disease? J Obstet Gynaecol Can 2014;36: 642–7.

71. Buchbinder A, Sibai BM, Caritis S, et al. Adverse perinatal outcomes are significantly higher in severe gestational hypertension than in mild preeclampsia. Am J Obstet Gynecol 2002;186:66–71.

72. Abalos E, Duley L, Steyn DW, et al. Antihypertensive drug therapy for mild to moderate hypertension during pregnancy. Cochrane Database Syst Rev 2018;(10):CD002252.

73. Magee LA, von Dadelszen P, Rey E, et al. Less-tight versus tight control of hypertension in pregnancy. N Engl J Med 2015;372:407–17.

74. Magee LA, von Dadelszen P, Singer J, et al. The CHIPS randomized controlled trial (control of hypertension in pregnancy study): is severe hypertension just an elevated blood pressure? Hypertension 2016;68:1153–9.

75. von Dadelszen P, Ornstein MP, Bull SB, et al. Fall in mean arterial pressure and fetal growth restriction in pregnancy hypertension: a meta-analysis. Lancet 2000;355:87–92.

76. Magee LA, Pels A, Helewa M, et al. Diagnosis, evaluation, and management of the hypertensive disorders of pregnancy. Pregnancy Hypertens 2014;4:105–45.

77. Magee LA. Drugs in pregnancy. Antihypertensives. Best Pract Res Clin Obstet Gynaecol 2001;15: 827–45.

78. Rey E, LeLorier J, Burgess E, et al. Report of the Canadian hypertension society consensus conference: 3. Pharmacologic treatment of hypertensive disorders in pregnancy. CMAJ 1997;157:1245–54.

79. Visintin C, Mugglestone MA, Almerie MQ, et al. Management of hypertensive disorders during pregnancy: summary of NICE guidance. BMJ 2010; 341:c2207.

80. Committee opinion no. 692: emergent therapy for acute-onset, severe hypertension during pregnancy and the postpartum period. Obstet Gynecol 2017; 129:e90–5.

81. Abalos E, Duley L, Steyn DW. Antihypertensive drug therapy for mild to moderate hypertension during pregnancy. Cochrane Database Syst Rev 2014;(2): CD002252.

82. Pickles CJ, Symonds EM, Broughton Pipkin F. The fetal outcome in a randomized double-blind controlled trial of labetalol versus placebo in pregnancy-induced hypertension. Br J Obstet Gynaecol 1989;96:38–43.

83. Lydakis C, Lip GY, Beevers M, et al. Atenolol and fetal growth in pregnancies complicated by hypertension. Am J Hypertens 1999;12:541–7.

84. Weber-Schoendorfer C, Hannemann D, Meister R, et al. The safety of calcium channel blockers during pregnancy: a prospective, multicenter, observational study. Reprod Toxicol 2008;26:24–30.

85. Cooper WO, Hernandez-Diaz S, Arbogast PG, et al. Major congenital malformations after first-trimester exposure to ACE inhibitors. N Engl J Med 2006; 354:2443–51.

86. Hecker A, Hasan SH, Neumann F. Disturbances in sexual differentiation of rat foetuses following spironolactone treatment. Acta Endocrinol 1980;95: 540–5.

87. Collins R, Yusuf S, Peto R. Overview of randomised trials of diuretics in pregnancy. Br Med J (Clin Res Ed) 1985;290:17–23.

88. Duley L, Meher S, Jones L. Drugs for treatment of very high blood pressure during pregnancy. Cochrane Database Syst Rev 2013;(7):CD001449.

Moving?

Make sure your subscription moves with you!

To notify us of your new address, find your **Clinics Account Number** (located on your mailing label above your name), and contact customer service at:

Email: journalscustomerservice-usa@elsevier.com

800-654-2452 (subscribers in the U.S. & Canada)
314-447-8871 (subscribers outside of the U.S. & Canada)

Fax number: 314-447-8029

Elsevier Health Sciences Division
Subscription Customer Service
3251 Riverport Lane
Maryland Heights, MO 63043

*To ensure uninterrupted delivery of your subscription, please notify us at least 4 weeks in advance of move.

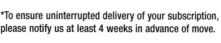